THE
WALKING
DIET

THE
WALKING
D I E T

WALK
BACK TO
FITNESS
IN
30
DAYS

LES SNOWDON AND MAGGIE HUMPHREYS

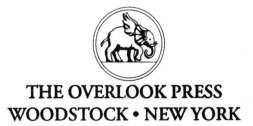

THE OVERLOOK PRESS
WOODSTOCK • NEW YORK

First published in the United States in1993 by
The Overlook Press
Lewis Hollow Road
Woodstock, New York 12498

Library of Congress Cataloging-in-Publication Data

Snowdon, Les
The walking diet : walk back to fitness in 30 days / Les Snowdon.
Maggie Humphreys.
p. cm.
1. Walking–Health aspects. 2. Physical fitness. 3. Reducing diets.
I. Humphreys, Maggie. II. Title.
RA781.65.S66 1993
613.7'176–dc20
92-35036
CIP
First published in Great Britain in 1991 by Mainstream Publishing
Manufactured in the United States of America on acid-free paper
Book design by Bernard Schleifer
ISBN: 0-87951-596-1
135798642

Walking is the best medicine
HIPPOCRATES

I have two doctors, my left leg and my right
G. M. TREVELYAN

*Not running, not jogging, but walking is your most
efficient exercise and the only one you can safely
follow all the years of your life*
QUARTERLY REPORT
— EXECUTIVE HEALTH ORGANIZATION, CALIFORNIA

*The land of our better selves is most surely reached
by walking*
H. I. BROCK

The longest journey starts with just one step
TAO TE CHING

CONTENTS

INTRODUCTION

Of all exercises walking is the best

THOMAS JEFFERSON

IN ONE SENSE YOU COULD SAY THAT WE BEGIN OUR LIVES IN THE wheelchair of the womb; we begin our lives literally by being carried around. In fact it would be true to say that many of us spend most of our lives being carried around.

As we leave the womb, enter the world and grow, and get over the initial wonder of walking, we change our prenatal wheelchair for a series of substitute wheelchairs—bicycles, motorcycles, cars, taxis, buses, trains, airplanes—and chairs (in houses, schools, offices; anywhere where people gather and sit).

For this is the age of "homo sedentarius" (sedentary man), the man who sits. In all ages prior to our modern scientific age, people had a more physical and active lifestyle. They spent more time on their feet than they did sitting.

But this is no longer true. Surveys show that nearly 60 percent of Americans don't get any regular exercise and 80 to 90 percent don't engage in regular aerobic exercise, which is the best way to keep the heart healthy. A report in *Prevention* magazine, February 1991, estimated that more than 22,000 people in New York alone might die during the year "clinging to their armchairs." And recent calculations by scientists at the U.S. Centers for Disease Control show that about 250,000 deaths a year in the United States can be attributed to a sedentary lifestyle.

In fact things are so bad that according to a report in *Circulation*, July 1992, The American Heart Association recently changed the status of physical inactivity from a "contributory factor" for heart and blood-vessel diseases and stroke to a "risk factor." This puts a sedentary lifestyle on a par with high blood cholesterol, high blood pressure and cigarette smoking.

And it's not just adults who have become increasingly sedentary. A 1992 Harris survey found that one-third of children between the ages of 3 and 17 were heavy for their age—a 42 percent increase over the previous seven years—and that 57 percent of children between 13 and 17 were overweight. Kenneth Cooper, M.D., M.P.H., president of the Cooper Aerobics Center in Dallas, Texas, said "children are becoming less active—they no longer walk or ride bikes to school—and television has given them more opportunities to be sedentary." Further surveys show that the average child watches between 15 and 25 hours of television each week.

Yet, for a time, it seemed there was evidence that this pattern was changing—that we were getting more active.

As the 1980s came to an end, the fitness movement worldwide had become a multi-billion dollar industry. People everywhere were "working out," "going for the burn" and driving themselves to keep fit. Punishing exercise routines became almost an alternative religion for many people. For the first time exercise had become an end in itself.

But, on reflection, the 80s were mostly about obsessional lifestyles, body consciousness, diet fads, work-out videos, designer leotards, designer shoes and designer water. Despite all the encouraging signs, the benefits of fitness seem as far away as ever, even for the declared enthusiasts. Marketing studies show that most home-gym equipment goes unused and 70 percent of Americans who own running shoes don't use them. Other surveys show that 60 percent of those starting jogging programs drop out or burn out within three months and that more than 40 percent of people attending aerobics classes sustain injuries which prevent them from exercising.

So the increased interest in fitness may not be the healthy trend that it first appeared to be.

EXERCISE—THE FINAL FRONTIER

For more than two decades now, first one, then another exercise program has been thrust at us as the answer to all the ills of modern living from heart attacks to stress. We have been preached to by film stars and eastern gurus; by so called fitness experts and by celebrities who want to tell us how to maintain youthful looks. Books on jogging, cycling, swimming, rowing, aerobics, and various exercise routines all crowd the bookshelves clamoring for our attention. Yet how many people who buy all these books are still actively following the exercise programs laid out in them?

And what have all these books been telling us to do?

TO JOG—Jogging is popular and many claim it is the best way to exercise. We have all seen the new jogger in a designer track suit and shoes, puffing and panting along the pavement, joints creaking and heart pounding as though his life depended upon it. But the truth is that it is easy to overdo jogging. Jogging has a high failure rate with beginners, and is the cause of numerous painful injuries. Ankle strain, foot strain, stress fractures, strained knee ligaments and inflammation of the Achilles tendon are all common injuries suffered by joggers.

TO SWIM—Swimming is a good form of exercise, but unless you have regular access to a swimming pool, it's unlikely that you will ever be able to swim enough to gain any real benefit from it. Another drawback is that water does not allow the full natural movement of the body under the force of gravity which is needed to develop and retain structural strength in the bones.

TO CYCLE—Cycling avoids the excess strain that running puts on the joints, but tends to overdevelop the leg muscles. Getting out in the open air on a bike can be an exhilarating experience. It is aerobic and helps build stamina but it is difficult and potentially dangerous in traffic; and like jogging it is easy to overdo. Stationary exercise bikes are no better, with the need for long periods of hamster-like moronic trundling to get any real benefits from them. Some people aim to do half an hour every day. Good luck to them. Ten minutes, in our experience, is enough to bore anyone out of his mind.

Other enthusiasts have been trying to persuade us to do aerobics—whether step-aerobics, dance-aerobics or whatever the next incarnation will be—as well as skip, row and a dozen other things to keep fit. Exercise and fitness has become the final frontier.

Whatever next?

Maggie and I were no different from anyone else. The 1980s had left us both with spreading waistlines and a feeling that we were beginning to slow down. Like many people around 40 we desperately needed a program for diet and exercise that would fit in with our busy lifestyles.

Yet we knew that if a program was going to work it had to be "user friendly"—we had had enough of diet and exercise books written by doctors and self-proclaimed experts. We did not have the time to visit the swimming-pool three times a week, and we were not interested in pumping iron or trundling around on an exercise bike every morning.

We had tried to combine exercise with a healthy diet. We both played tennis and squash and most weekends we would walk in the countryside, on the hills or along the seashore. We had tried cycling, skipping and jogging and we each had an exercise bike in the spare room. But like many people we had sustained injuries and we had finally become disillusioned about ever becoming fit.

We felt that our diet was reasonably balanced. We had increased our fiber intake and we were eating more fish, fruit and vegetables. We had reduced our consumption of saturated fats, sugar, salt and alcohol. Neither of us smoked. And yet despite all this the pounds were creeping up on us and we seemed to be fighting a losing battle.

So what were we doing wrong?

Quite simply, like millions of other people, we had become sedentary. We were spending too much time sitting.

"But hold on," we can hear you say, "I thought you said that you walked on weekends and played tennis and squash."

True. But that still makes us sedentary, like most other people. For if you are not exercising aerobically using some form of whole body continuous movement (brisk walking, jogging, cycling) for 30 minutes at least three to four times a week, then by definition, you are sedentary.

Let's say you spend 15 minutes sitting down for breakfast. Then you spend another 30 minutes sitting in a car (the average driver spends nearly two weeks each year sitting behind the wheel), bus or train on the way to work. When you arrive at work you may then spend at least another six hours sitting in a chair working. Then 30 minutes back home again and about another four hours sitting around the house before going to bed.

Is this an exaggeration?

Not for many people it isn't. And if you think about it, that's more than 11 hours each and every weekday. And unless you make a special effort to do something active on a weekend, then you can add another 16 hours or so to the total, making a grand total of more than 70 hours each week.

If you exclude the eight hours on average spent in bed each night, then you could be spending around 65 percent of your entire waking life in one form of sedentary position or another. You could be described as being no more than a brain on wheels or a brain stuck in a chair.

And don't say that you are much more active than the people described above, for the sedentary label applies to most people in Western society, including club golfers, club squash and tennis players, mailmen, and Mrs. Smith next door who is out in all weather walking her dog. The figures for the percentage of sedentary people at the beginning of this chapter tell only part of the story.

Being active is not enough!

If you are not regularly stretching your body aerobically in some form of continuous whole body exercise, then you are sedentary.

Join the ranks of homo sedentarius—you have a problem.

WALKING—THE BEST EXERCISE

These men I have examined around the world who live in vigorous health to 100 or more years are great walkers. If you want to live a long, long time in sturdy health you can't go wrong in forming the habit of long vigorous walking every day... until it becomes a habit as important to you as eating and sleeping.

DR. LEAF,
EXECUTIVE HEALTH ORGANIZATION, CALIFORNIA

Experience tells us that many people who take up jogging, cycling, and other aerobic routines often sustain injuries, or simply give up after a short time. They join the increasing number of people who regularly try to get fit and fail.

So what are they doing wrong?

There are only two facts you need to know about exercise:

1. IF YOU DON'T DESIGN AN EXERCISE PROGRAM FOR YOURSELF THAT REMAINS ENJOYABLE AS YOUR FITNESS IMPROVES YOU'LL QUIT!

That is why it is often only enthusiasts who are still cycling, swimming, jogging and doing aerobics. The rest of us quit a long time ago.

2. EXERCISE REALLY MEANS CONTINUING TO EXERCISE: TODAY, TOMORROW AND FOR THE REST OF YOUR LIFE.

Exercise is not a short-term cure like taking an aspirin to cure a headache. If exercise is to be effective it must become as natural to us as breathing, eating, or cleaning our teeth. Otherwise most of our efforts are all a waste of time and energy.

This is why walking scores every time:

- Walking is the best exercise—it is a totally natural activity; your enjoyment will improve as your fitness improves.
- Walking is habit-forming; the more you do it the more you will want to do it.
- Walking aerobically will give you all the fitness benefits of jogging, cycling and dance aerobics—without the injuries.
- Walking aerobically makes you slim and is the perfect weight-management system.
- Walking is simple and safe; just about anyone can do it, including the young, elderly and those recovering from illness.
- Walking is a prevention against heart and circulatory disorders and may lower blood pressure.
- Walking will help you to sleep and is an antidote to stress, nervous tension and depression.
- Walking can improve your posture and may prevent lower back pain.
- Walking requires no special skills or equipment.
- Walking can be done almost anywhere.

Regular, vigorous aerobic exercise like brisk fitness walking can lead to beneficial physiological changes in many of the body's processes: lower blood pressure, lower cholesterol level, and improved cardiovascular and respiratory response.

Many of the benefits that come from brisk walking are due to the CV effect—the effect produced on the cardiovascular (CV) system. By gently stretching the capacity of the heart and lungs through exercise, the CV system's capacity is increased. This is what makes this type of exercise (like jogging and cycling) aerobic.

But if exercise is not kept up, the body reverts to its original inactive state. Former athletes who stopped exercising were found to have the same risk factor for a heart attack as those who had never been active. It can take three to six months of regular vigorous aerobic exercise to build up a powerful heart and lungs; and it can take the same period of inactivity to lose it all.

I began serious fitness walking after the long hot summer of 1989. For the first time in my life I had a weight problem. I had put on about 15 pounds during the year and I was beginning to take on the traditional pear shape. My waist size had suddenly increased and I could not get into my trousers any more.

I was determined to lose the weight. I had always loved walking so it seemed the obvious thing to do. I would simply get out more often and walk faster and for longer.

I decided on a 30-day plan. I felt that if I could get into a regular habit-forming routine then I would be able to keep it up beyond the 30 days. My plan was to increase my pace from normal (around 3 miles per hour) to brisk (3.5–4.0 miles per hour) and to walk longer and further as the weeks went by. And the key to maintaining the regularity and discipline would be to walk out of my front door and do a circuit around the block and back home again. I knew that if I had to drive to the park or into the country first, then the walking would never get done except on weekends. This was the key to the whole thing: REGULAR, RHYTHMIC BRISK WALKING OUT OF MY FRONT DOOR, AROUND THE BLOCK AND BACK AGAIN.

After two weeks I felt better and I had lost several pounds. Although previously I had been walking only on weekends, I was now walking up to five times a week for half an hour at a time. I was not only losing weight but I felt better: fitter, more alert, more energetic.

The plan was working.

After 30 days of aerobic fitness walking and cutting down on foods that were high in fat, I had walked away 7 pounds. I was able to get back into some of my trousers and I was well on the way to my ultimate goal of health and fitness.

Maggie had also started to use the plan and walk her way to health and fitness. We both knew that walking alone would not keep the pounds off forever. We had to get our diet right also.

Maggie has always loved cooking and everything to do with food, so she began to put together all her low-fat recipes, and a complete diet/exercise program evolved which would not only get rid of the pounds but keep them off forever.

And so The Walking Diet evolved.

The one thing that we decided from the outset was that calorie counting was out. We couldn't seriously go on counting calories all our lives. No one can, or should. What we needed was a moderate approach that we could work with—*live with*.

The ancient Greek concept of diet had impressed us both. To them "diata" meant a way of living, a way of finding wholeness through health, fitness and correct nutrition.

This had to be the way to go. With regular brisk walking, and eating the right kinds of food, we can be fit and healthy without having to resort to extreme, fanatical exercise routines or brutal, calorie-counting diets.

Our own experiences with walking were very quickly confirmed when we read in *Newsweek*, November 1989, that after the most detailed fitness study ever carried out by the Aerobics Institute, it had been established that moderate exercise can have all the beneficial effects that are normally associated with hard, "no pain, no gain" exercising (see Table 1).

The *Newsweek* report confirmed that moderate brisk walking for half an hour three to four times a week is all

Table 1

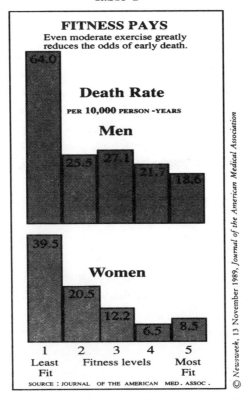

FITNESS PAYS
Even moderate exercise greatly reduces the odds of early death.

Death Rate

PER **10,000** PERSON -YEARS

Men

64.0
25.5
27.1
21.7
18.6

Women

39.5
20.5
12.2
6.5
8.5

| 1 | 2 | 3 | 4 | 5 |
| Least Fit | | Fitness levels | | Most Fit |

SOURCE : JOURNAL OF THE AMERICAN MED . ASSOC .

© *Newsweek*, 13 November 1989, *Journal of the American Medical Association*

that is needed to provide protection not only from cardio-vascular disease and cancers, but also against death from a wide range of other causes. A study at the Centers for Disease Control in Atlanta found that the least active people were almost twice as likely to have heart disease as those who were most active. A further study at the University of Utah Medical School showed that men who exercised moderately and expended just 1000 calories a week in exercise had 30 percent less chance of developing heart disease than those who were sedentary.

But one of the largest studies of all was The College Alumni study of 17,000 Harvard graduates, carried out over a period of 20 years by Dr. Ralph Paffenberger of

Stanford University. He found that those who exercised regularly were fitter and tended to live longer and were "significantly less likely to suffer a heart attack than were their sedentary classmates." The study also demonstrated that "by age 80 those who exercised regularly could expect to add one or two years to their lives." And it was walking that was the most popular exercise reported.

Fitness walking is at the heart of a revolution which is changing the entire way that people view fitness and health. Since the early 1980s, fitness walking has grown in the United States from an infant activity to being the largest participant activity for people of all ages—and that includes jogging and aerobics.

According to the National Sports Goods Association, fitness walking shows the fastest growth among all fitness activities—up 60 percent in less than five years, from 41.5 million participants to 66 million (1991 survey).

When we developed The Walking Diet, we had no idea that it was soon to become the fitness success story of the 90s.

THE WALKING DIET SUCCESS STORY

The Walking Diet was launched in April 1991 and within weeks it was on the bestseller lists throughout Britain and Ireland. After a nationwide publicity tour throughout the United Kingdom, the book had its Irish launch in Dublin on Pat Kenny's late night TV talk show, "Kenny Live." A politician, Jim Kemmy, an actress, Eileen Coghan, and two members of the audience, Teresa Corrigan and Julie Stapleton, all volunteered to be weighed, and to go away and do The Walking Diet.

When the Walking Dieters returned to his show five weeks later, the ebullient Pat Kenny said: "After the last show the book walked off the shelves; it was No. 1 in the bestsellers."

Pat Kenny, a great walker himself, then weighed the dieters, and the results were astonishing. Jim Kemmy, who was very overweight, had lost 42 pounds; Julie Stapleton, 17 pounds; Teresa Corrigan, 14 pounds; and Eileen Coghan, 9 pounds.

When Pat Kenny interviewed us initially, and asked how much weight the participants could all expect to lose, we had said that a good target was to aim for about 1–2 pounds a week. Eileen Coghan had done this easily, but her fellow dieters proved what can be done when you really set your heart on something. Not only did they lose weight, but this is what they said about walking:

Eileen Coghan: "I'd recommend it to anybody. I feel as fit as a flea and toned up. I sleep better—like a top—and I have more energy. I loved it, I feel great and I'm going to keep it up."

Teresa Corrigan: "The walking was excellent. After a week you felt so good, much fitter with endless energy. You wanted to get up in the mornings and get going."

Julie Stapleton: "I loved the walking. I had great energy. After the first week I really enjoyed it."

And this is what Jim Kemmy said after losing his 42 pounds on The Walking Diet: "It's a good guide. It gives you the motivation, but it's up to you basically."

It's up to you basically. It is. But with a little help, guidance, and motivation from us, you also can join The Walking Dieters above and feel great...feel fitter...have endless energy...be toned up...sleep like a top...be dying to get out of bed in the mornings...and lose—well that's up to you!

As far back as 500 B.C. the founder of modern medicine, Hippocrates, was telling people that "walking is the best medicine." Now, in the 1990s, more than forty scientific studies have shown that moderate exercise such as fitness walking is the best way for people of all ages to get fit and stay fit for life. Combined with a healthy eating plan—the walking diet—fitness walking is the easiest way to keep fit and shed those unwanted pounds and keep them off forever.

Everywhere, "homo sedentarius" (sedentary man) is giving up his inactivity to become "homo ambulans" (walking man). It is now official. Not only is fitness walking the best, cheapest, all-round exercise available to everyone young and old, but it is "green" and natural. The Walking Diet is *the* diet exercise of the 1990s.

·1·

DIATA—A
BETTER WAY
OF LIFE

The first wealth is health

RALPH WALDO EMERSON

- In the United States this year 1.5 million people will have heart attacks
- In the United States this year 500,000 people will die from a heart attack
- In the United States this year heart disease will be the No. 1 killer of men over 40
- In the United States this year 500,000 people will die from cancer
- In the United States this year, 180,000 women will learn that they have breast cancer—that is nearly one every three minutes

By anyone's standards these statistics are alarming and are at epidemic proportions. The United States vies with Sweden and Russia for top heart-attack nation, and since the 1950s heart disease has killed more Americans than anything else. And the United States has the highest incidence of breast cancer in the world.

25

But it's not just heart disease and cancer that are the problem. Americans are just as prone to other "Western diseases." Diabetes, hemorrhoids, varicose veins, mental illness, arthritis and tooth decay all play their part in reducing the quality of life for large numbers of people each year.

There is now considerable evidence of a link between diet and exercise and the extent to which they influence the risk of disease. Diet has been clearly implicated in two of the major factors in the development of heart disease— elevated cholesterol and high blood pressure. Scientists now estimate that 30 percent of all cancer incidence is related to diet. And according to the United States Surgeon General, of the 2.1 million Americans who die each year, 1.5 million, 68 percent, die from diet-related diseases.

These problems are not restricted to life in the United States and the rest of the Western world. No matter where one looks throughout the world, wherever a Western sedentary lifestyle coincides with a Western-style diet, the above effects can be observed. We are what kills us.

CHANGING TIMES

The better off we are, the more energy-rich, dense calorie foods we eat: meat, cheese and chocolate. And we eat more convenience foods, which are high in calories: cakes, cookies, pastries, pizzas, burgers, potato chips and other snack foods. In the United States, about 200 people every second order at least one hamburger and on a typical day 45 million people eat in fast food restaurants.

In contrast to modern man, prehistoric man, "homo erectus," was a hunter-gatherer, walking through necessity, and running to pursue and capture his prey. He had a high fiber diet and plenty of exercise. Modern man, however, homo sedentarius, does not need to pursue his food. Every type of food is readily available and preparation and cooking have never been easier; and if he cannot spare the time, convenience foods reduce the time required for shopping and preparation to the bare minimum.

But we do not have to go back to prehistoric times to witness the change in our diet. Most of the changes have taken place in the past 200 years and many in the past 50 years.

We keep animals in pens to fatten them. Homo sedentarius, in contrast, does not need to be kept in pens. He accepts voluntary inactivity and as a result gets fat.

It has been observed that some people switching from using a typewriter to a personal computer can gain up to 7 pounds a year because they no longer have to get up to consult filing cabinets; and the same effects can be observed when people use remote-control television, extension phones, elevators and dishwashers.

And consumption of foods tends to be higher in sedentary people; as a result they tend to have lower metabolic rates than active people and an increased chance of becoming even fatter.

Since the end of the Second World War Americans have been getting fatter. 40 percent of women and 20 percent of men are obese by middle age. It is estimated that between the ages of 20 and 60 a sedentary woman gains about 27 pounds. This is because as we get older we tend to become more sedentary (less active) and our metabolic rate slows down. We seem to be forever "fighting the flab," going on crash diets, and trying to cut calories.

Yet essentially, we are what we eat. During the 20th century the average person in Western society has been eating too much fat and too little fiber. A hundred years ago the average person ate less than 25 percent fat in their diet; today half our energy is derived from fat in different forms. That is bad news for our figures and bad news for our health.

"YOU CAN'T GET FAT EXCEPT BY EATING FAT!" (Martin Katahn, *T-Factor Diet*)

The former United States Surgeon General, Dr. C. Everett Koop, commented recently that FAT IS WESTERN SOCIETY'S GREATEST NUTRITIONAL HAZARD. Is it any wonder then that the Western way of eating is also the Western way of dying?

There are no simple answers as to why people suffer from cardiovascular, respiratory, and other Western diseases. But various characteristics of population and lifestyle are usually blamed for the problem:

- Poor diet
- Lack of exercise
- Family history
- Obesity
- Stress
- High blood pressure
- High cholesterol level
- Alcoholism
- Smoking

All of the available evidence on lifestyle and nutrition suggests that by eating a healthier diet, exercising regularly, and finding time for relaxation, many of the above problems can be reduced if not eradicated. And a moderate approach to alcohol and the cutting out of smoking would save needless deaths and improve the quality of people's lives.

DIET AND DISEASE

Diet and disease are inseparable. You would think from the figures for deaths and illness from Western diseases that little was being done to improve the situation.

You would be wrong.

Health education and nutritional information are widely available to everyone. Newspapers and magazines carry extensive coverage of diet and health topics and diet books are among the bestsellers. In 1990 more than 25 new diet books were launched and the market is increasing. If you add to this the growing number of health and fitness-related books then you would expect us all to be getting healthier and fitter.

And we are trying to become healthier. A survey released in November 1990 suggested that 90 percent of us are trying to eat more healthily. This follows on from the 1970s and the health conscious 80s when increasing numbers of people were becoming more responsible towards themselves and their lifestyle.

Yet despite all the good intentions, health and fitness for large numbers of people are still elusive goals which seem to be getting further and further away. According to a survey by the Calorie Control Center, 48 million Americans were on diets in 1991.

People are genuinely trying to become more health conscious and fit. A 1989 Gallup Fitness Consumer Survey found that women are not only using diets and exercise to improve their looks but also their health.

For many people the problem of how to become fitter and healthier is more a question of method than intention. And that is where "diata" can help.

DIATA

Eating is about making choices; healthy eating is about making the right choices. And like exercise, it's all about balance and moderation. It's no use going on extreme reducing diets this week if we end up giving them up next week. We need something we can work with today, tomorrow and the rest of our lives.

Healthy eating is about much more than the kinds of food we eat. It's also about lifestyle, which affects eating habits. We like to think of it in terms of the ancient Greek idea of "diata" which means literally "a way of living." It is both how we exercise and what we eat that defines our "diata."

Diata suggests a holistic way of looking at our health and lifestyle to find a balance and rhythm that is lacking. When you think about it the ancient Greeks had some pretty good ideas. The motto engraved on the wall of the temple at Delphi was "Know Thyself," and was adopted by the philosopher Socrates as the basis for the study of philosophy. It is also the basis for "diata." Know yourself: know your own body and mind; know what your real needs are.

To listen to many authorities on nutrition, you might think that eating is an exact science. Having analyzed the calories in every type of food under the sun, they then try to organize your entire life around their rigid schedules, telling you exactly what to eat and what to avoid.

The truth is that eating is not an exact science and never will be. How many people consciously buy food each week in an organized, scientific way? Eating is not a science; it is an art. It is much more a question of knowledge and awareness of which foods to eat and which to avoid than it is of following blindly someone else's strict regime.

Knowledge, awareness, and the desire to change are the best motivations you can have. This is what diata is: a balanced, moderate approach which will provide the long-term benefits that you desire.

The biggest single change you can make in your lifestyle is to do a personal food and drink audit—an awareness audit of what you eat and drink. Write down a list of everything that you regularly eat and drink, and compare it with the following recommended lists of foods and drinks to increase and decrease. This will enable you to work out the changes you need to make in your diet and plan your own personal "diata."

PERSONAL FOOD AUDIT

Increase your consumption of:

OILY FISH

herring, sardines, tuna, trout, salmon, bluefish, mackerel, shad, redfish, pompano

WHITE FISH

cod, haddock, sole, turbot, monkfish, grouper, halibut, shark, tilefish, red snapper, pike

VEGETABLES

potatoes, carrots, peas, cabbage, tomatoes, cauliflower, broccoli, Brussels sprouts, spinach, green beans, parsnips, onions, leeks, eggplant, zucchini, garlic, sweet corn, asparagus, bean sprouts, celery, cucumber, bell peppers (green/red/yellow), radishes, green onions, Belgian endive, lettuce, fennel, watercress

GRAINS AND LEGUMES

beans, chickpeas, lentils, bread (whole grain), rice (whole grain), pasta, cereals (whole grain), bran, seeds, nuts, oat bran

FRUIT

apples, pears, oranges, bananas, grapefruit, lemons, limes, pineapple, guava, passion and other exotic fruits, mango, nectarines, apricots, grapes, berries, melon

Decrease your consumption of:

SATURATED FATS

meat and meat products: beef, pork, lamb, sausages, bacon, liver, burgers, luncheon meat, liver sausage (replace with lean cuts of red meat; chicken, turkey, game); dairy products: whole milk, cream, butter, cheese (replace with: skim milk, low-fat yogurt, low-fat cheeses)

VEGETABLE OILS/FATS
palm oil, coconut oil, lard (replace with small amounts of sunflower, safflower, corn & soy and canola oils, olive oil, polyunsaturated margarine spreads)

SNACKS

potato chips, peanuts, other packaged snack foods

REFINED CARBOHYDRATES

sugar, chocolate, desserts, cookies, pastries, puddings, pies, white bread, rolls, crackers

SALT

PERSONAL DRINK AUDIT

Increase your consumption of:

WATER

6 to 8 8-ounce glasses daily

(Water is our most important nutrient; up to three-quarters of the body's weight is water. It regulates body temperature; assists all bodily functions.)

ANY LOW-CAL SOFT DRINK

Decrease your consumption of:

ALCOHOL

maximum: 3 units per day for men
2 units per day for women
1 glass of wine, 1 beer, 1 shot of hard liquor, each equal one unit)

Alternate with low-alcohol/alcohol-free drinks with food; drink with an equal measure of water; try two or three AFDs— alcohol-free days—each week; cut out altogether, if desired.

COFFEE

Drink weaker, without milk, or with 2% or skim milk; try decaffeinated.

TEA

Try weak Darjeeling or any other tea, or herb or lemon tea, or try decaffeinated tea.

A NEW BALANCE

A good diet should maintain health, provide energy, promote growth, and give protection against disease.

Here are the American Heart Association's main dietary recommendations:

1. Total fat intake should be less than 30 percent of daily calories
2. Saturated fat intake should be less than 10 percent of daily calories
3. Carbohydrate intake should make up 50 percent or more of daily calories, with mostly complex carbohydrates
4. Protein intake should provide the rest of the daily calories

The important thing to remember is that we should all be seeking to eat more of the right kinds of food (foods with health and nutritional properties) rather than seeking to fit in with someone else's ideal consumer. Using the personal food and drink audit we should be seeking a new balance in our diet that will provide us with all the essential nutrients that our bodies need.

We need nutrients for energy, cell growth, organ function, and efficient food utilization. The six important nutrients are carbohydrates, proteins, fats, vitamins, minerals and water. Macronutrients (carbohydrates, protein and fat) need micronutrients (vitamins and minerals) to release the energy contained in them. During digestion, enzymes then break these nutrients down so that they can be absorbed through the walls of the digestive tract and enter the bloodstream.

Using the Personal Food and Drink Audit, Walking

Dieters will be provided with all the essential nutrients that they need. Water has already been covered in the audit; fats, proteins and carbohydrates are covered below in the section "Where to Begin." Now just a few words about vitamins and minerals.

Vitamins are natural substances vital for growth and health. They cannot be manufactured by our bodies. Some are needed for the efficient action of enzymes; others form essential parts of hormones. The most important thing to know about them is that they work synergistically with minerals: that is, they enhance each other, adding up to more than the individual sum of their parts. We need them all.

There are water soluble and fat soluble vitamins. Water soluble vitamins are the range of B vitamins (B_1, B_2, B_3, B_5, B_6, B_{12}) and vitamin C. The B vitamins are found in the staple foods (whole grain bread, brown rice, oat bran, nuts, grains) and meat, fish, eggs, milk, poultry, green vegetables, bananas and cheese. Vitamin C is found in green, leafy vegetables, potatoes, tomatoes, fruits and berries.

The B vitamins are often called the "stress vitamins." They are essential for a healthy nervous system and they give protection against infection, aid in energy production and promote growth. Vitamin C is also required by those under stress and by smokers, and it is important for the growth and repair of cells, gums, blood vessels, bones and teeth. And it helps in healing disease.

Both B and C vitamins, being water soluble, cannot be stored in the body and must be replaced daily. However, the fat soluble vitamins—A, D, E and K—can be stored in the body and these can be found in root vegetables, spinach, cheese, milk, eggs, fish, fish oils, dairy foods, nuts, green vegetables, and cereals. They promote growth, give protection from infections, and are essential for other body functions.

The important minerals are calcium, zinc, iron, potassium, magnesium, phosphorous and iodine. Other minerals required by the body are selenium, manganese, sodium, and other trace elements. Like vitamins, they cannot be manufactured by the body, so they must be provided in our daily diet. They can be found in milk, cheese, soy beans, seafood, poultry, green vegetables, meat, eggs, nuts, beans, seeds, oat bran, citrus fruits, apples, bananas, and potatoes.

New research suggests that we should eat more foods rich in the "ACE" vitamins—beta-carotene (a form of vitamin A), vitamin C and vitamin E. All three are known as anti-oxidants, which neutralize destructive chemicals called "free radicals" which can promote diseases like cancer and heart disease. Doctors at Harvard Medical School also believe that anti-oxidants present in beta-carotene may reduce the effects of LDL, or "bad cholesterol." (See information about cholesterol in next section.)

Where to find them -

BETA-CAROTENE:
dark green leafy vegetables, yellow and orange vegetables and fruits such as spinach, broccoli, peas, watercress, asparagus, carrots, sweet potatoes, tomatoes, apricots, peaches, cherries, mangos, cantaloupe
VITAMIN C:
citrus fruit, strawberries, kiwi fruits, raw cabbage, green leafy vegetables (as above), green peppers, potatoes, parsnips, tomatoes
VITAMIN E:
nuts, seeds, whole grains, soy beans, vegetable oils (especially sunflower oil), fish liver oils, green leafy vegetables

Three good portions of vegetables and two of fruit each day is the best way to ensure that you get enough of the "ACE" vitamins.

36

If you follow The Walking Diet you will get the vitamins and minerals that you need. However, anyone who is on the move, under stress or is likely to skip meals should think about taking a multi-vitamin and mineral supplement to make up for any deficiencies in diet. Remember that the B vitamins and vitamin C cannot be stored in your body. They need replacing every day.

WHERE TO BEGIN

Start by Reducing Fat

Each fat gram that you eat contains 9 calories. Each protein and carbohydrate gram you eat contains 4 calories. It is the fat in your diet that makes you fat. Our bodies are designed to burn carbohydrates and store fats.

The important thing is not to count calories, but to recognize those foods which are fat-dense. It is fat-awareness, not calorie-awareness, that is needed.

The main thing to cut is saturated fat which can cause high blood cholesterol levels, leading to clogged up arteries and potentially a heart attack or stroke.

At present most Americans get between 35 to 40 percent of their total daily calories from fat—and 15 to 20 percent of those calories are from saturated fat. We have already noted that on a typical day 45 million Americans eat in fast food restaurants. And it has been estimated that between 40 and 55 percent of calories in most fast food meals come from fat, mostly in the form of saturated fat, which helps to raise cholesterol levels.

Saturated fat is found in foods of animal origin such as red meat, butter, milk, cheese and cream. Use skim milk, margarine low in saturated fats, low-fat cheese, reduced calorie mayonnaise and low-fat yogurt instead of cream.

And try to avoid frying food wherever possible, cutting out fat, and using an oil for cooking which is low in saturated fat and high in polyunsaturates—sunflower, corn, canola, and soy oil.

The body actually needs fat. In order to grow and function effectively, fat is needed by the brain, muscles, heart, hair, skin, immune system, and cell walls, etc. The problem is that we have got the balance wrong. What we need is an oil change!

Research done among the Greenland Eskimos has shown that they have almost no record of heart disease. This is because the key factor in their diet is the amount of seafood they eat daily. Seafood contains Omega-3 fatty acids. These particular fatty acids can play a significant role in preventing heart disease and clogged up arteries. High levels of these fish oils can be found in mackerel, herring, sardines, tuna, trout and salmon.

Research recently carried out by the Medical Research Council in Cardiff involved 2,033 men under 70 who had suffered a heart attack. One group of men was told to eat foods rich in Omega-3 fatty acids at least twice a week. After two years it was found that the fish eaters had up to 30 percent less chance of dying from a second heart attack than those who had been told nothing about fish.

Fat from a land-based diet is known as Omega-6. The best advice now available is to cut down on Omega-6 fats and balance them with Omega-3 fish oils.

A word about cholesterol. Cholesterol has had a bad press. Although it can be responsible for a variety of illnesses, it is actually essential for health.

It is present not only in the bloodstream but in all of the body's tissues. Most of the cholesterol in the blood-stream is made in the body, but some foods which we eat contain cholesterol (dietary cholesterol).

Cholesterol is transported in the blood by lipoproteins.

There are two types of lipoproteins—high density lipoproteins (HDLs) and low density (LDLs). HDLs are sometimes called "good" and LDLs "bad" cholesterol. The higher your HDL level the lower the risk of heart disease.

You can affect your total cholesterol level through your diet. Dietary cholesterol is only found in foods of animal origin—in meat, eggs and dairy products. As a diet high in cholesterol and saturated fat can increase your blood cholesterol level, it is essential to reduce your intake of cholesterol and saturated fat.

It is interesting to note that Eskimos have higher HDLs than those of us eating a typical Western diet. This is due to their larger consumption of Omega-3 fatty acids which contain the polyunsaturated fats EPA (eicosapentaenoic acid) and DHA (docosahexoenic acid). The other beneficial effects of these fish oils have already been observed above.

A recent study at the USDA Human Nutrition Research Center on Aging at Tufts University shows that good cholesterol is now even better. Their findings show that even if your total cholesterol is in the safe range (less than 200), low levels of HDL are dangerous—it is the balance of HDL and LDL that is more critical than the total amount of cholesterol. These findings were based on research into heart attack victims, 34 percent of whom had low levels of HDL. New guidelines recommend aiming for a HDL level of over 40, with some experts suggesting that 50 should be the goal.

The National Institute of Health estimates that about 40 million Americans have cholesterol levels high enough to require attention. The best way to lower total cholesterol and to boost HDL levels is to make lifestyle changes—particularly diet and exercise. Following The Walking Diet—by cutting saturated fat and eating more fish, white meat, complex carbohydrates, fruits and vegetables, and walking aerobically four times a week for thirty minutes—is the best way to boost HDL levels.

Several studies in the United States have suggested that aerobic exercise like fitness walking can increase HDL levels as much as 10 to 20 percent. And according to the British exercise physiologist Dr. Adrianne Hardman of the University of Loughborough: "Regular walking can increase the levels of 'good' cholesterol in the blood, reducing chances of a heart attack." She claims that exercise is the best lifestyle change you can make to increase your HDLs.

Stress can also affect your cholesterol level. When you are stressed, sugar from the liver is released into the bloodstream to provide extra energy for the muscles, and there may also be an excessive release of cholesterol. So try to avoid stress—and relax. Go for a fitness walk.

It has also been observed that moderate alcohol drinkers (two glasses of wine, beer or whisky a day) have higher levels of HDLs in their blood; so it seems that a bit of alcohol each day may actually be good for you.

Reduce Refined Carbohydrates

Carbohydrates, along with fats and proteins, are one of the three main building blocks of life. Carbohydrates are compounds of carbon, hydrogen and oxygen and their function is to provide energy. There are two types: simple and complex, or sugar and starches.

Simple carbohydrates are digested quickly, while complex ones are digested slowly, which means they can provide more energy and stamina. Some carbohydrates in a Western diet, such as sugar and syrup, are refined and provide little food value.

Sugar has been described as "pure, white and deadly."

The average American consumes 133 pounds of sugar a

year, which accounts for about 20 to 25 percent of calories—500 to 600 calories per day per person! It provides energy but hardly any nutrients. If we cut it out of our diet today we will be none the worse off but will have a head start in reducing our total intake of calories.

But remember, sugar does not only come out of a packet. Two-thirds of our annual consumption is hidden in processed foods such as cakes, cookies, beer and soft drinks. Even some brands of breakfast cereal contain up to 25 percent sugar. Almost all canned foods contain sugar. So watch the labels.

Eating refined carbohydrates such as those above can raise the blood cholesterol level, and is a possible cause of heart disease.

Other refined carbohydrates, such as white flour and white rice, like sugar, have been stripped of most of their vitamins, minerals and fiber content and should be replaced with unrefined staple foods such as listed in the Personal Food Audit.

Reduce Protein

Proteins are divided into two types: animal and vegetable. Animal protein, or first class protein as it is known, contains all eight essential amino acids which the body depends on for good health. Vegetable protein, or second class protein, lacks some of these amino acids, the one exception being soy beans.

In our Western diet we eat more than twice as much protein as we need, and of an unhealthy type. We should cut down on red meat, always choose lean cuts and eat more white meats, such as chicken and turkey. We should also eat more fish. Fish is an excellent, low calorie source of protein. Four ounces of cooked white fish provides one third of our total daily requirements for less than 100 calories. Fish is also a rich source of vitamins and minerals which the body needs, and we have already seen above the benefits obtained by eating fish containing Omega-3 fatty acids.

As long as all the amino acids are present, all protein is ultimately the same. If legumes are combined with nuts and grains, or seeds (sunflower, pumpkin, sesame, etc.) then the body should be under no risk of protein deficiency. But people who wish to reduce animal protein by including some vegetarian dishes in their diet may wish to include eggs but in a limited way, as they are high in cholesterol. Eggs are the perfect protein, containing all eight essential amino acids, so they can make up for any deficiency that may be caused elsewhere.

Increase Fiber

Fiber helps you lose weight, and we should be eating at least 30 grams a day of it. Fiber is found in complex carbohydrates which consist of starches and fiber bound up together in such things as bread, potatoes, fruit, vegetables, nuts and beans.

Fiber is important to us in healthy eating because it provides filling food without being fattening. Bulky carbohydrates satisfy our hunger with less than half the calories weight for weight of fatty food: 1 gram of carbohydrate is 4 calories; 1 gram of fat is 9 calories.

There are two types of fiber—soluble and insoluble. Insoluble fiber is found in cereals and in fibrous fruit and vegetables. This fiber, or roughage, helps food and waste products to pass through the digestive system. Food containing insoluble fiber is satisfying, as it needs more chewing than other foods and, as it absorbs water and swells in the stomach, it is filling.

Soluble fiber, found in fruit, vegetables and beans, helps

prevent hunger between meals, as it delays the absorption of certain nutrients. Without this fiber, there can be a large drop in the blood sugar level, which causes hunger. Oat bran, which is the outer protective coating of the oat grain, is one of the best sources of soluble fiber and can be eaten raw or cooked.

Inexpensive, pocket-size fat and fiber counters are available at any bookstore and they are a worthwhile investment in your good health. The following lists give a general idea of high and low fiber contents in some of the main foods:

HIGH

Peas Bran Prunes Beans
Sweet Corn Bananas Whole grain bread
Brown rice Dried fruit
Potatoes, baked and eaten with skin Leafy vegetables

MEDIUM

Most green vegetables Most nuts
Apples Oranges Celery

LOW

Potatoes, boiled White bread
White rice Tomatoes Lettuce
Cucumber Grapefruit

NONE

Meat Fish Eggs Sugar
Milk Butter Cheese

Reduce Salt

We eat up to ten times the amount of salt we actually need; on average about two teaspoonsful a day, half of which is added by manufacturers during food processing.

Too much salt can cause high blood pressure, which can increase the risk of heart disease. If you eat a balanced diet you will get all the salt you need without having to add it to your diet. Try reducing your use of salt slowly over a period of weeks and use flavoring substitutes like herbs, spices and lemon juice. Try to break the habit of adding salt at the table, if necessary using a low sodium salt substitute. And cut down on potato chips, snack foods and canned foods.

A WAY OF LIFE

In a recent survey carried out for *New Woman* magazine, 500 women between the ages of 20 and 45 were asked about their personal experiences of losing weight. The majority claimed that the best method for them was simply cutting down on fattening foods, and following healthy eating habits. The report concluded that "all the evidence is that while a gradual change in eating patterns may yield slower results, those results are far more likely to prove permanent."

The Walking Diet is not a short term cure. It is a long term solution to fitness and health. Walking makes you slim, builds cardiovascular fitness, and can develop into a long term habit that you can use for the rest of your life. And your own personal "diata" will help you to build up the long term eating habits that are necessary for good health.

We have suggested that "diata" means a way of living;

it means taking a holistic viewpoint on the food we eat and the exercise our bodies need. It means taking into account our current eating habits and including in our diet the necessary changes that are required to maintain a healthy lifestyle.

Don't let anyone tell you that diet and exercise don't go together. THEY DO. A balanced healthy approach to lifestyle (your own personal "diata") is a balance between healthy eating, exercise and relaxation.

AND DON'T FORGET! Homo sedentarius is most of us: your spouse perhaps, your father, Uncle Fred, the family next door, the girl sitting all day behind the reception desk at work.

Don't become next year's statistics. Switch off the television set, follow the recipes, get out and walk, and just LET GO. Remember, your health is in your own hands; or should that be feet?

·2·

WALKING
MAKES YOU
SLIM

*If you do not get active and stay active,
you've got a snowball's chance in hell
of maintaining any weight loss. You
will face semi-starvation for the rest
of your life if you remain sedentary and
want to control your weight.*

MARTIN KATAHN, THE ROTATION DIET

Millions of people have already discovered the magic of walking and are walking regularly for fitness, slimness and health. Why cause ourselves so much anxiety, and spend so much time, money and energy on failed diet/exercise routines when the answer to all our problems is staring us right in the face.

Walking is the easiest, cheapest, most convenient, most effective (in the long term) exercise of all. And we have been doing it all our lives. The only problem is that we are not doing enough of it and in the right way.

To begin with we already have a solid foundation from which to build our exercise program. We all walk a certain amount every day of our lives, even if we are sedentary, and that is easier than starting from scratch for the first time jogging or cycling.

Our bodies already use the muscles required to walk, so it is simply a question of increasing the duration and then the intensity of our walking in order to build up to the fitness level that we require.

But it is still boring old walking, isn't it?

No, it isn't.

Forget about strolling down to the shops to get a newspaper or sauntering in the park with the family on Sundays. For that is exactly what it is, strolling and sauntering. There is nothing wrong with that. Both activities can be very enjoyable. But neither activity will get you very far in your quest for fitness, and to be honest they give walking a bad name.

Brisk fitness walking—aerobic walking—is an exhilarating experience. Aerobic walking provides all the fitness benefits of jogging, cycling, and rowing with less chance of injury, "burn-out" and sheer boredom. And it really does make you slim.

HOW IT WORKS

There was a time when diet books insisted that exercise could not help in losing weight. But these days most experts agree that regular whole body continuous exercise, such as brisk fitness walking, is a necessary part of a successful weight loss program.

And it works for several reasons:

1. IT'S AEROBIC—The key to walking aerobically is to walk at a pace of 3.5–4.0 miles per hour for a minimum of 20 minutes, during which time the heart rate is elevated to 60–80 percent of its maximum. Below 60 percent the exercise will not have an aerobic effect and only very fit people can gain any aerobic effect above the 80 percent level (see Table 2).

Table 2

AGE	MAXIMUM HEART RATE	60% LEVEL	80% LEVEL
20	200	120	160
25	195	117	156
30	190	114	152
35	185	111	148
40	180	108	144
45	175	105	140
50	170	102	136
55	165	99	132
60	160	96	128
65	155	93	124
70	150	90	120

If you think about it, air is essentially the "breath of life." We cannot live without it, but many of us are living each day with too little of it. Our sedentary lifestyle induces shallow breathing and instead of inhaling as much as 3,000 cubic centimeters of air, we often inhale as little as 500 cubic centimeters. Imagine what the performance of your car would be like if you reduced the air supply to the carburetor. It would jump and shudder and you would have a very uncomfortable ride. Lack of sufficient oxygen affects our bodies in the same way. We feel tired and sluggish and cannot be bothered to do anything. We are trying to run our bodies on too little air.

Aerobic means literally "with oxygen," and walking aerobically causes the lungs to take in more air with less effort. The lungs are then able to extract more oxygen from the increased air supply and deliver it to the cells where it is needed to combine with food to produce energy.

It is this increase in oxygen that provides the extra fuel to burn up the food in our internal fire. When oxygen is supplied to a flame it burns faster; the same thing happens to our body when we walk aerobically. The action of the lungs works like a bellows which enriches the internal fire where food is converted into energy. The result is an improvement in the vital efficiency of the lungs and the whole cardiovascular (CV) system.

As the CV system improves, the blood vessels enlarge and become more elastic, and the heart becomes bigger and stronger. The muscles are strengthened by an increased flow of blood, as are the ligaments that attach them to the bones. Strength and mobility of joints improves, and because the muscles need more energy, stored body fat is broken down and utilized, leading to a reduction in weight.

It is the heart and lungs that help to determine the fitness of the whole body. Other organs, although vital in their own way, cannot survive without a blood supply rich in oxygen and nutrients. Whenever you run for a train, cope with stress at work, or lose your temper, the heart and lungs have to cope with the extra demands placed on them. Your heart beats faster; your lungs take in more air. And it is the healthy CV system that can cope easily with all the strains placed upon it by modern living. Conversely, it is the weak CV system that is easy prey to high blood pressure, coronary attack, colds, viruses, and other diseases. Listen to what Gabe Mirkin and Martshall Hoffmann in *The Sportsmedicine Book* say about the athlete's heart:

Because the athlete's heart is so muscular it can pump the same amount of blood with 50 beats per minute that the average heart pumps with 75 beats. Thus the athlete's heart will beat 13 million fewer times per year. It works less, rests more, and consequently takes a much longer time to wear out.

You may not end up with an athlete's heart through aerobic walking, but you will have gone a long way to improving its strength and efficiency, thus ensuring a longer and healthier life.

You should now be able to see that aerobic walking is vigorous sustained exercise that provides all the health and fitness benefits of jogging, cycling and rowing. And it is this regular aerobic routine that speeds up the body by increasing its metabolic rate and gives it the ability to shed those extra pounds.

2. IT INCREASES YOUR METABOLIC RATE—Aerobic exercise such as brisk, fitness walking speeds up your metabolic rate. Basal or resting metabolic rate (BMR) is the speed your body burns calories at rest—in other words carrying out the job of staying alive: blood circulation, cell growth, digestion, thinking and so on.

The BMR of a man or woman is dependent on weight, height, fitness and body composition. Body composition is the amount of lean muscle compared with fat. A fat 150-pound person will have less lean tissue in total body mass than a thin 150-pound person, the difference being the excess fat.

A person's total daily need for calories is the amount of calories needed to maintain BMR plus the calories needed for movement, i.e. physical activity. Everyone's BMR is different. The important thing is that we can influence it through aerobic exercise.

The problem of dieting without increased physical activity is that the BMR slows down rather than speeds up. Then when you stop dieting, the body, which has been acting in a kind of starvation mode, finds that it has become used to its new BMR and requires less calories to function. And so it deposits the extra calories it does not need as fat. Dieting without exercise also forces the body to manage on less oxygen, and it reduces its oxygen intake even further when it has to take energy, not from food, but from the body itself.

In contrast, during aerobic walking the heart and respiratory rates increase and the BMR speeds up. It is the increase in oxygen and the increased BMR that burns off excess calories and keeps them off forever.

Generally speaking, compared with being sedentary (sitting watching TV, working at a desk), you will burn around three times more calories walking at 3 miles an hour. And when you walk aerobically at 4 miles an hour, you will burn around five times more calories than you would being sedentary.

Table 3 is an estimate of the calories you can expect to burn off as you increase your activity from a gentle stroll to brisk aerobic walking. It is based on a person weighing 150 pounds. These figures are only estimates because people have different metabolic rates. Men normally have higher BMRs than women because a larger part of their total body weight is muscle tissue, and muscle tissue can burn up to three times more energy than fat tissue, even when it is inactive.

Aerobic walking will help change your body composition by increasing the amount of muscle tissue compared with fat tissue. This is important because up to half the weight normally lost on calorie-reducing diets without exercise is muscle tissue. And this loss of muscle tissue lowers BMR rather than increases it.

This is the problem of dieting without exercise. You can end up losing weight, lowering your BMR and be stuck with maintaining a semi-starvation diet to keep the pounds off. Regular aerobic walking, on the other hand, will increase your BMR and still allow you to eat well and stay healthy and slim.

Increased BMR is good news for aerobic walkers. For not only does it burn off on average up to 100 calories for every 15 minutes of activity, but the raised BMR can continue to burn off calories for several hours after exercis-

Table 3

WALKING SPEED M.P.H.	PACE	CALORIES BURNED (APPROX.)	
		IN 30 MIN	IN 1 HOUR
2	SLOW	120	240
2.5	MEDIUM	140	280
3	MEDIUM	160	320
3.5	BRISK	180	360
4	BRISK	210	420
4.5	FAST	250	500
WALKING UP MODERATE INCLINE	BRISK	300	600

ing is over. And there is evidence to suggest that sustained aerobic walking not only increases BMR but that the increased BMR continues permanently.

3. IT SHEDS FAT—Most diets are calorie based and rely on calorie restriction for results. Until recently it had always been assumed that all calories are the same, regardless of where they came from. In other words a fat calorie was exactly the same as a carbohydrate or a protein calorie. And if we over ate on any one of them then any surplus energy would end up by making us fat. However, recent research has confirmed that all calories are not the same.

Studies at Stanford University and at the Human Nutrition Center in Maryland have overturned the conventional wisdom. In one research study a group of overweight women were given a high fat diet while another group received a low fat diet. Both provided the same amount of calories. It was found that women on the high fat diet gained weight more easily than women on the low fat diet and a similar project for men reached the same conclusion.

The Vanderbilt Weight Management Program has produced similar results. Martin Katahn confirms that "it's the fat in your diet that makes you fat... when it comes to being fat and overweight, it's primarily the fat calories that count, not the carbohydrate and protein calories" (*T-Factor Diet*).

In the typical Western diet all the energy in protein is burned up daily and none is converted and stored as fat. And whereas protein and carbohydrates use 25 percent of energy converting dietary fat to body fat, fat itself requires very little energy to convert dietary fat to body fat—3 percent in fact. It is the ease with which the body converts dietary fat to body fat that causes the main problem in weight control. It is not just weight control that we need but fat control.

Although the body is not as efficient at converting excess carbohydrate to body fat as it is at converting dietary fat to body fat, it was thought until recently that any extra calories would still end up as body fat. This has now been disproved. Under most circumstances the body converts very little carbohydrate to body fat. Our bodies are designed to burn carbohydrates and store fats.

And this is where metabolic rate (BMR) comes in again. Because if you eat a regular high carbohydrate diet then your BMR is likely to be higher than a person eating a high fat diet. Your body has to work that much harder to convert the additional carbohydrate into energy and it is this thermic effect (the thermal factor, or T-factor) which can burn off up to another 200-300 calories each day. And remember that this is in addition to the calories you are burning away every day during aerobic walking, another 200-400 calories depending upon time and effort.

The thermic effect (thermogenesis) is the action of the body in burning up excess calories consumed as food energy to produce heat. The additional thermic effect produced by The Walking Diet (low fat food and aerobic exercise) will gradually help produce the change in body shape that you desire and bring you back to your target weight.

As we know, exercise plays an important part in any diet/exercise routine, but the key thing is that all exercise is not the same. Aerobic walking carried out as part of The Walking Diet will burn off more fat during the activity period than carbohydrate. Not only will you burn off up to 300 calories walking briskly at 4 miles an hour for 45 minutes, but up to 180 of these calories will be fat calories.

In contrast, if you perform an anaerobic (literally "without air") activity such as squash for 45 minutes, then you will burn off up to 650 calories but only about 260 of these will be fat calories. This is because regular continuous aerobic exercise like brisk walking is a fat burning activity whereas start-stop anaerobic exercises like squash and tennis are carbohydrate burning activities.

During aerobic walking your heart and breathing rates increase, level out, then remain there for the duration of the exercise. Your body is supplied with the oxygen it needs when it needs it to burn in its fuel mixture. Anaerobic exercise on the other hand requires short sudden bursts of energy which are provided by fuel supplied from the muscles, and not from the increased oxygen supply provided by aerobic exercise. This leads to the feeling of rapid heart beat and breathlessness that is typical of anaerobic exercise.

The good news for everyone is that aerobic walking has the greatest effect around the hips and thighs where fat tends to accumulate, particularly in women. This is good news for all women who have been unsuccessful with hip and thigh diets that concentrate mainly on dieting and calorie-counting. It's also good news for men who are trying to lose weight around their hips and thighs and especially their waistlines. Regular aerobic activity not only burns off this excess fat, but it keeps it off forever.

I hope you are now convinced that regular aerobic walking is the answer to all your exercise and diet needs and that you cannot wait to get out and try it. As the saying goes, the journey of a thousand miles begins with just one step, so by now you should be thinking of putting all your good intentions into practice and getting out to walk.

STARTING OUT

This walk is the beginning of a habit which will change the rest of your life. So put on suitable clothing and a pair of comfortable sturdy shoes and set yourself a target of a 20 minute brisk invigorating walk.

You can walk almost anywhere that is convenient and safe, but we have found that the easiest and quickest way to build a regular walking habit is to walk right out our own front door and do a circuit around the block and back again. Once you start walking regularly you can vary your walks by going to the park, the beach or the hills. But in the beginning you should make it as easy as possible to get into the habit without excuses getting in the way. The aim is to start walking and keep walking.

But first a HEALTH WARNING!

If you are uncertain about your physical condition; if you are overweight, suffer from cardiovascular or respiratory disease, or have a medically diagnosed problem, then you should consult your doctor before starting to walk briskly. And beware of the passive fitness syndrome. Just because you are thin and never suffer a day's illness does not mean that you can embark on an energetic walking program without building up to it. The advice is always the same. Warm up first (follow the exercises in Chapter 4—The Walker's Workout), start slowly and don't hurt yourself, for that is the fastest way to break the routine in your program and is often the reason why so many exercise programs fail.

The resting pulse rate (heart rate) is a rough guide to your general physical condition. It is a barometer which determines your state of well-being, stress or illness. It should be taken first thing in the morning, before it has had time to be increased by exertion, mental excitement, eating, or stimulants like tea, coffee or nicotine.

Take your resting pulse rate by first sitting quietly in a chair and breathing normally. Then use either of the following methods:

1. Place the first two fingers of your right hand on the main artery of the inner wrist of your left hand just below the base of the thumb. Count the number of beats in either

15 or 30 seconds and multiply by either four or two to obtain the resting pulse rate.

2. Place two fingers on your neck beside your windpipe; you will feel the pulse. This is the carotid artery which carries blood to the head. Count the number of beats in the same way as for the wrist. Whatever you do, don't press both sides of the neck at the same time: you could diminish the flow of blood to the head, or even cut it off.

Your pulse rate changes throughout the day. It is lowest while sleeping. On awakening it will rise from five to ten beats a minute, and during the day it will rise gradually and may be up to ten beats higher at bedtime than it was when you got up in the morning.

Pulse rates vary greatly. Generally speaking, the lower the resting pulse rate, the healthier you are. The average for men is between 70 and 85 a minute; a woman's pulse tends to be faster at 75–90 beats a minute. If your pulse rate is between 90 and 100, it is likely that you are unfit, and a brisk walking routine will gradually bring it down. Having said that, some people have normal pulse rates up to 100 and some athletes and other normal people have pulse rates as low as 40. The main thing to remember is that the heart is simply a pump: the less work it has to do (the fewer beats it makes), the longer it is going to last.

You should now begin your walking routine to suit your physical condition. If you have been sedentary for some time and are not used to physical exertion, then you should begin slowly, walking for no more than 20 minutes every other day, at a pace which stretches you but does not overtire you. Your goal should be to exert yourself a little more each time until you reach a brisk pace and you feel comfortable with it. On alternate days walk at a slower pace to help you build up a regular habit of walking. Then continue walking at this pace until you feel ready to go on to the 30 day walk back to fitness program given later in this chapter.

Whatever you do don't hurt yourself. It is at the beginning of an exercise routine, when the desire for results exceeds the ability to cope, that you will suffer from musculo-skeletal injuries. It's at this point that so many people give up. The beauty of walking is that no matter where you start, you can gradually build up the duration and intensity of your routine until you reach the fitness level that you require.

If you are already physically active, then you should start out with a brisk, vigorous walk for 20 minutes, stretching yourself as you walk. At the end of it you should feel refreshed. If you feel tired then you are going too fast. If you cannot hold a conversation with someone without getting out of breath then you are going too fast. The key to the whole thing is to listen to what your body is telling you and to slow down if necessary. You should walk briskly every other day, and on alternate days walk for 20 minutes at a slower pace to build up a regular routine, until you feel ready to go on to the 30-day walk back to fitness program at the end of this chapter.

To get the real benefits of aerobic walking and to walk towards that fitter, slimmer you, you have to achieve a walking heart rate between 60 percent and 80 percent of your maximum heart rate (refer again to Table 2).

There is a simple way of calculating your aerobic walking rate. Subtract your age from 220. This gives your maximum heart rate in beats per minute. Then multiply that figure by 0.60 (60 percent) for the lower end of your aerobic walking rate and by 0.80 (80 percent) for the higher end.

After you have been walking for about ten minutes take your pulse. You will need a watch that records seconds for this. Take your pulse in the same way that you calculated your resting pulse rate earlier. If your heart is beating beyond the high end of your aerobic range then you are walking too fast. If you are unfit, three miles an hour will probably be a comfortable rate to walk at to reach your aerobic range.

When you first start out you should stick to the lower end of your aerobic range (60 percent) until you feel comfortable with it. Then as you progress, measure your aerobic improvement by taking your pulse at several points during the walk and immediately upon finishing. This will ensure that you remain within your aerobic range.

As your fitness improves you will find that your heart rate decreases while performing the same level of exercise. This is because the increased size and strength of the heart muscle enables it to pump a larger volume of blood into the arteries with each beat.

Once you are comfortable walking at the 60 percent level, then experiment up to the 70–75 percent level. You should not need to go higher than this. At this level you should get all the fitness, slimness and cardiovascular benefits that you need.

But as you progress from the 60 percent level upwards, remember that your body is the best judge of what feels comfortable. If it hurts then slow down. Gentle stretching is what is needed, not painful exertion. There is nothing more demoralizing than coming home with an injury which keeps you out of action for a few weeks.

WALKING WITH THE WEATHER

You should keep up your walking routine regardless of the weather. There are few days when the weather is so unpleasant that it is impossible to walk; and even on a rainy day there are often periods when the rain stops. After all, the weather does not normally stop you getting to work, playing golf, or getting on with the rest of your life.

On a cold day you can keep your whole body warm with far less clothing than you may think. The main thing is to wear gloves, cover your head and neck, and keep your thighs warm. When the extremities are warm, the whole body can be kept warm with light clothing. If you start to feel too warm you can always take off the hat and gloves.

Don't put on too many sweaters. Instead, wear several light layers of clothing that can easily be added or removed as you walk. There are some excellent lightweight clothes available these days made from such materials as Gore-Tex, which keep out the wind and rain but allow your sweat to evaporate.

For warm-weather walking, wear light-colored clothes to reflect the heat and light, and if it is sunny, wear a brimmed hat. Choose a time of day such as early morning, late afternoon, or early evening to walk.

Don't let the weather put you off. Once you build up a regular routine you will want to get outside whatever the weather is doing. And remember that you are walking for the psychological benefits as well as the fitness and slimness benefits. Each season has its own delights to offer. Mist and fog, snow, spring rain, and summer heat are all attractive and beautiful to the walker who takes the time to look.

FINDING YOUR STRIDE

Pace is the key to finding your stride and reaching a good rhythm in your walking. Set off at a good pace with the longest stride that is comfortable, letting your arms swing naturally in opposition to your feet.

The arms should move at the same speed as the legs. Relax your shoulders, then as you walk the arms will swing by themselves. When your right foot swings forward, your left arm will swing with it; when your left foot swings forward, your right arm will swing in opposition to it. The arms and shoulders move and swing in a pendulum motion in counterbalance to the legs and hips.

The legs and hips have the largest muscles in the body: let them set the rhythm, then let the arms follow that rhythm. You will notice that as your legs speed up so do your arms. Your elbows will bend naturally and you will feel the natural flow of brisk rhythmic walking.

With each stride you will begin to feel yourself reaching further with your hips. This is good news! The more you stretch your hips the more you will improve your shape. If you continue to stretch your hips forward, you will find that they move naturally without any sort of exaggerated wiggle.

You will now want to make sure that your feet are landing in the right place. The most comfortable and efficient way is to use the heel-toe method. The heel of your leading foot should touch the ground, just before the ball of the foot and toes. Then, as the heel touches the ground, lock your ankle and shift your weight forward with the knee bent, rocking forward onto the toes and using them to push you off to the next step.

WALKING TO YOUR GOAL WEIGHT

The first thing to do is to find a pair of old jeans or other piece of favorite clothing that is too tight and use this as a measure for making progress. There is nothing like the thrill a week or two later of being able to get back into clothing that you thought had been discarded forever.

Next, weigh yourself and make a note of it. If you don't know your height then measure that too. Then check yourself against the Height/Weight Chart (see Table 4). For each height there is an acceptable weight range covering small to large frames. If you are a woman your goal weight should be nearer the lower figure; for men, depending on build, it should be towards the higher end of the scale.

You now have a goal to aim for. But don't get obsessed with weight watching. Body weight fluctuates rapidly at times. Weigh yourself once a week and try to get back into your chosen piece of clothing. If you build up an aerobic walking program you will soon see the excess pounds drop away and you will feel and look fitter and slimmer without weight watching.

Table 4

Height and Weight Tables

	Women		
Height	Small Frame	Medium Frame	Large Frame
4'10"	102-111	109-121	118-131
4'11"	103-113	111-123	120-134
5'0"	104-115	113-126	122-137
5'1"	106-118	115-129	125-140
5'2"	108-121	118-132	128-143
5'3"	111-124	121-135	131-147
5'4"	114-127	124-138	134-151
5'5"	117-130	127-141	137-155
5'6"	120-133	130-144	140-159
5'7"	123-136	133-147	143-163
5'8"	126-139	136-150	146-167
5'9"	129-142	139-153	149-170
5'10"	132-145	142-156	152-173
5'11"	135-148	145-159	155-176
6'0"	138-151	148-162	158-179

NOTE: Weights at ages 25 to 59 based on lowest mortality. Weight in pounds according to frame (in indoor clothing weighing 3 pounds, shoes with 1-inch heels).
SOURCE: Courtesy of Metropolitan Life Insurance Company Statistical Bulletin.

	Men		
Height	Small Frame	Medium Frame	Large Frame
5'2"	128-134	131-141	138-150
5'3"	130-136	133-143	140-153
5'4"	132-138	135-145	142-156
5'5"	134-140	137-148	144-160
5'6"	136-142	139-151	146-164
5'7"	138-145	142-154	149-168
5'8"	140-148	145-157	152-172
5'9"	142-151	148-160	155-176
5'10"	144-154	151-163	158-180
5'11"	146-157	154-166	161-184
6'0"	149-160	157-170	164-188
6'1"	152-164	160-174	168-192
6'2"	155-168	164-178	172-197
6'3"	158-172	167-182	176-202
6'4"	162-176	171-187	181-207

NOTE: Weights at ages 25 to 59 based on lowest mortality. Weight in pounds according to frame (in indoor clothing weighing 5 pounds, shoes with 1-inch heels).

SOURCE: Courtesy of Metropolitan Life Insurance Company Statistical Bulletin.

By now you should have been out on several practice walks and determined your state of fitness. You should be listening carefully to what your body is telling you and you should be judging your pace and duration so that you finish tired and refreshed, not exhausted.

You are now ready to make some real progress. But don't look for instant results. Concentrate rather on the walking itself. Get into the habit first of feeling the sheer thrill and exhilaration of getting out of doors away from telephones, noise, and distractions. Think about how good you feel. Tell yourself that this is a habit which is going to change your life forever, and that it is going to bring you the health, fitness and slimness that you deserve.

I promise you that if you persevere with aerobic walking the psychological benefits alone will make you want to get out every day. So let yourself go. You are learning to do the most natural thing in the world. This is what your body was designed for.

DISTANCE, TIME AND SPEED

As we have stressed previously, the easiest way to begin aerobic walking is to walk out of your own front door and do a circuit round the block and back, or around some other convenient route that is known to you. You will need to gauge the distances covered so the best way is to take a car ride around your proposed route and use the odometer to measure the distance between familiar landmarks. Alternatively, some bicycles have an odometer on them which you could use in the same way.

As you build up your walking program, you will need to increase the length of your circuit if you are going to cover several miles. And you will need to measure it. Or you can simply cover as many circuits as you want around the same track in the way that athletes do circuit training on a track. And you will want to calculate your speed.

It is useful to remember the following formulas:

1. Distance = Speed x Time

2. Speed = $\dfrac{\text{Distance}}{\text{Time}}$

3. Time = $\dfrac{\text{Distance}}{\text{Speed}}$

If you know any two of the above variables, it is easy to work out the third. Time is the easiest to measure: most people have a watch. So if you can measure the distance, it is then easy to calculate the speed.

Once you begin to stray from easily measured routes and landmarks, you will need to acquire a pedometer. A pedometer is a small gadget that clips onto your belt and you adjust it to the length of your own stride to measure the distance covered. With the help of your watch, it will also tell you the speed at which you are traveling. Pedometers can be purchased in most sports shops and large department stores.

There are two further methods to estimate the distance covered while walking:

1. WALKING SPEEDS (M.P.H.)—Walk for one mile along the route you have previously measured with the car's odometer and time yourself. If it took you 15 minutes then you were walking at 4 m.p.h.:

$$\text{Speed} = \frac{\text{Distance}}{\text{Time}} = \frac{1 \text{ mile}}{0.25 \text{ hours}}$$

As you vary your walking pace (increase your speed), then repeat the above method to calculate your new walking speed. You will soon get a feel for the speed you walk at and be able to judge different walking paces (2.5, 3.0, 3.5, 4.0 m.p.h.). If you can estimate your speed, and you know the time, then it is easy to work out the distance:

Distance = Speed x Time

2. THE STEP METHOD—Count the number of steps that you take in one minute at your normal walking speed. Since the average stride is approximately two feet per step

and there are 5,280 feet in one mile then it will take 2,640 steps to cover one mile. If your speed is 176 steps per minute then it will take 15 minutes to cover one mile:

Distance = Speed x Time
        = 176 steps/min x 15 mins
        = 2,640 steps

You may want to measure your exact stride in the way that a pedometer does. To do this, measure the distance from toe to toe or heel to heel when you take a normal stride. The easiest way is to get someone to help you. Then calculate the distance walked in the same way as above.

All this may sound very complicated. It is. The easiest way to measure distance is to get hold of a pedometer.

WALK BACK TO HEALTH & FITNESS IN 30 DAYS

At the same time as you begin your 30 day walking program, you should also begin the 30 day Walking Diet as detailed in Chapter 3. You should be aiming to lose 1-2 lbs. per week until you get back to your goal weight. This is quite enough to lose, and it is the most efficient way to control weight loss. It is quite normal of course to have a rapid weight loss of several pounds in the first week due mainly to water loss (our bodies are 70 percent water).

Although the walking program and the diet routine are organized through Day 1 to 30, we recommend that you begin the program on a Monday, as the aerobic walking gradually builds up throughout the week, with more aerobic walking on weekends.

Before you walk, always warm up first (using the warm-up exercises in Chapter 4—The Walker's Workout). Then start slowly, and build up your speed as you go along.

As this chapter proceeds, there is an aerobic walking record for you to fill in. If you wish, you can copy this and use it as an ongoing walking record after the 30 days. The record will help to measure your progress and to motivate you; for it is motivation that will get you going, and it is motivation that will keep you going. If you keep this up to date, then you can plan each day or week in advance, inserting where, when and for how long you are going to walk. You will notice that each day is divided into a.m. and p.m. Some days you may not be able to fit in your daily walk in one session, so you can divide it into an a.m. and a p.m. session. However, we do not recommend that you split the times for your aerobic walks during the first 14 days. Walk for 20 or 30 minutes aerobically, as directed, during this time, either a.m. or p.m. Then, if you wish, split your walks into a.m. and p.m. on alternate days when you are walking at a moderate pace.

The times suggested throughout the 30 day program are minimum times that you should walk each day. If you hit your stride and get a rhythm going, you may feel comfortable going on a little longer than the minimum times. If it feels good, then go a little further before finishing. Then as you walk each day you can compare your actual, achieved time against your planned time; and you can record the distance, speed and any other information about the route (whether it is flat, rough ground, or uphill). At the end of each week you can then add up your total time and compare your planned and achieved time to measure your progress; and you can do the same thing at the end of 30 days.

Please don't treat your walking record as a chore to fill in every day. Be businesslike about it. Clearly defined aims and objectives will bring you the results you desire, and remember: if you don't know where you are going, then how are you going to know when you arrive?

WEEK 1

DAY 1 - Begin by walking aerobically (3.5–4.0 m.p.h.) for 20 minutes around the route you have measured out. Start off at a good pace, with the longest stride that is comfortable, your arms swinging naturally in opposition to your legs. Remember to take your pulse at intervals along the walk to make sure you are within your aerobic range.

DAY 2 - Walk for 20 minutes at a moderate pace and simply take in the joy of walking. For the first three weeks you will be alternating aerobic walking with moderate walking for the first four days each week, followed by one day's rest. This will help you get into the habit of regular walking without placing too much emphasis initially on results.

DAY 3 - Walk aerobically for 20 minutes. Concentrate on finding your stride and building a good rhythm.

DAY 4 - Walk for 20 minutes at a moderate pace. You will now be feeling the psychological as well as the aerobic benefits of regular walking. You will not be able to wait to get out each day.

DAY 5 - Rest day.

DAY 6 - Walk aerobically for 20 minutes. As we have stressed, the times quoted are minimum times. Weekends are a good time to get in those extra miles and get away from your measured route— into the country, etc.

DAY 7 - Repeat Day 6. At the end of the first week you will have a solid foundation on which to build in future weeks. You will already be feeling fitter, healthier, and be starting to shed the first few pounds of excess weight.

		Time Planned (Mins)	Time Walked (Mins)	Distance In Miles	Speed In M.p.h.	Route/Comment
DAY 1	A.M.					
	P.M.					
DAY 2	A.M.					
	P.M.					
DAY 3	A.M.					
	P.M.					
DAY 4	A.M.					
	P.M.					

	Time Planned (Mins)	Time Walked (Mins)	Distance In Miles	Speed In M.p.h.	Route/Comment
DAY 5 A.M.					
DAY 5 P.M.					
DAY 6 A.M.					
DAY 6 P.M.					
DAY 7 A.M.					
DAY 7 P.M.					
WEEKLY TOTALS				Av. Speed	

71

WEEK 2

DAY 8 - You are now starting to make progress, and can increase your walking time from 20 to 30 minutes each day. The important thing is to increase time before pace; so walk at a moderate pace for 30 minutes, gently stretching yourself as you go.

DAY 9 - Walk aerobically for 30 minutes. It normally takes the first ten minutes of any brisk walk to get into a rhythm and feel aerobic, so increasing the time from 20 to 30 minutes is effectively doubling the aerobic benefits.

DAY 10 - Walk at a moderate pace for 30 minutes. Try early evening walks to de-stress after a hard day's work. Feel the rhythm in your feet, calves, thighs, arms and shoulders. Relax—and go with the flow.

DAY 11- Walk aerobically for 30 minutes. Think about the calories you are burning up—200 for every 30 minute walk!

DAY 12- Rest day.

DAY 13- Walk aerobically for 30 minutes. Remember that you are not only burning up calories while you walk, but your increased metabolic rate will keep burning up calories when you finish walking.

DAY 14- Repeat Day 13.

WEEK 3

DAY 15 - The cumulative benefits of regular walking will now be starting to add up and you will be well on your way to that healthier, slimmer you. You can now increase your walking time from 30 minutes to 45 minutes per day: walk at a moderate pace for 45 minutes. Take your spouse, a friend, or the children for a walk.

DAY 16 - Walk aerobically for 45 minutes. If you wish, split your walking time between a.m. and p.m. You can now start venturing away from your measured route and start looking for additional ways to clock up extra miles—try walking when doing errands instead of driving; try parking the car further away from work and walking the rest of the way; or getting off the bus or train one of two stops from your destination and walking the rest of the way.

DAY 17 - Walk at a moderate pace for 45 minutes. Think of all the opportunities that are available each day to walk, instead of taking the easy option by using cars, buses, taxis and trains. The miles all add up.

DAY 18 - Walk aerobically for 45 minutes. In your aerobic walking record we mentioned that you should make a note of conditions around the route. This is important because walking uphill requires more energy than walking along a level surface. Uphill walking is a greater calorie burner (up to 600 calories an hour); even rough road surfaces help to burn off more calories. Try small hills first.

DAY 19 - Rest day.

DAY 20 - Walk aerobically for 45 minutes. Try energy breathing as you walk: breathe in through the nostrils counting 1 to 8 then out through the mouth counting 1 to 8.

DAY 21 - Repeat Day 20.

		Time Planned (Mins)	Time Walked (Mins)	Distance In Miles	Speed In M.p.h.	Route/Comment
DAY 8	A.M.					
	P.M.					
DAY 9	A.M.					
	P.M.					
DAY 10	A.M.					
	P.M.					
DAY 11	A.M.					
	P.M.					

74

		Time Planned (Mins)	Time Walked (Mins)	Distance In Miles	Speed In M.p.h.	Route/Comment
DAY 12	A.M.					
	P.M.					
DAY 13	A.M.					
	P.M.					
DAY 14	A.M.					
	P.M.					
WEEKLY TOTALS					Av. Speed	

75

		Time Planned (Mins)	Time Walked (Mins)	Distance In Miles	Speed In M.p.h.	Route/Comment
DAY 15	A.M.					
	P.M.					
DAY 16	A.M.					
	P.M.					
DAY 17	A.M.					
	P.M.					
DAY 18	A.M.					
	P.M.					

		Time Planned (Mins)	Time Walked (Mins)	Distance In Miles	Speed In M.p.h.	Route/Comment
DAY 19	A.M.					
	P.M.					
DAY 20	A.M.					
	P.M.					
DAY 21	A.M.					
	P.M.					
WEEKLY TOTALS					Av. Speed	

WEEK 4

DAY 22 - Only nine more days to go. Today, walk at a moderate pace for 45 minutes. Vary your walking routine with morning walks, lunchtime walks, late afternoon walks, early evening walks. Try walking breaks instead of coffee breaks. The miles all add up.

DAY 23 - Walk aerobically for 45 minutes. Over the past week you have been walking away a minimum of 300 calories a day during your walk, and your increased metabolic rate will have been burning up another few hundred calories when you have finished walking. And all this is in addition to the calories you will be shedding by using the low-fat recipes in The Walking Diet

DAY 24 - Walk aerobically for 45 minutes. See the world at 4 miles an hour; this is what your body was designed for.

DAY 25 - Repeat Day 24. Cultivate awareness: savor the sights and sounds of the journey. Walk to break out of the pattern and routine of normal daily living.

DAY 26 - Rest day.

DAY 27 - Walk aerobically for 45 minutes. Try inner walking and walking meditation (see Chapter 6). Discover who you are. Walk for the inner benefits as well as the fitness and slimness benefits.

DAY 28 - Repeat Day 27.

DAY 29 - Almost there! Only two days left. Walk aerobically today for 45 minutes. After four weeks of aerobic workouts, you have built the foundations for a lifetime's health and fitness.

		Time Planned (Mins)	Time Walked (Mins)	Distance In Miles	Speed In M.p.h.	Route/Comment
DAY 22	A.M.					
	P.M.					
DAY 23	A.M.					
	P.M.					
DAY 24	A.M.					
	P.M.					
DAY 25	A.M.					
	P.M.					

		Time Planned (Mins)	Time Walked (Mins)	Distance In Miles	Speed In M.p.h.	Route/Comment
DAY 26	A.M.					
	P.M.					
DAY 27	A.M.					
	P.M.					
DAY 28	A.M.					
	P.M.					
WEEKLY TOTALS					Av. Speed	

80

	Time Planned (Mins)	Time Walked (Mins)	Distance In Miles	Speed In M.p.h.	Route/Comment
DAY 29 A.M.					
P.M.					
DAY 30 A.M.					
P.M.					
MONTHLY TOTALS				Av. Speed	

81

DAY 30- The final day: walk aerobically for 45 minutes. Feel the wind in your hair, and the satisfaction of a task well done. In the past 30 days you have been training your body to work at its optimum potential; and you will now have a good idea of what you can achieve by using The Walking Diet recipes and aerobic walking. Keep walking!

It may take longer than 30 days to achieve your goal weight; it depends how much you need to lose. But when you do achieve it, you will find that you can then use aerobic walking as part of an ongoing maintenance program to keep you at your goal weight. In future you will be in control of your own body.

Once you have reached your goal weight, you will want to maintain the health, fitness and slimness benefits that you have achieved. You should continue to walk aerobically for a minimum of 30 minutes each day, four times a week; and you should continue to use the low fat Walking Diet recipes and adapt them to your own diet.

Everyone binges on food from time to time, particularly at Christmas and holiday periods, but you will find that once aerobic walking becomes an enjoyable habit, it will be easy to walk away those excess pounds any time you need to. You simply use The Walking Diet, put your foot down, and clock up the necessary aerobic miles to get you back to your goal weight.

·3·

THE
WALKING
DIET

"Will you walk a little faster?"
said a whiting to a snail

LEWIS CARROLL

The recipes in The Walking Diet are easy to follow and quickly prepared, so that even the busiest people have a chance to cook mouth-watering food that is full of goodness and at the same time is low in fat.

Having formed the habit of buying lots of fresh fruit and vegetables, fish, white meat and low fat alternatives to dairy products, we need to cook interesting and attractively presented dishes. This is not difficult, even for an inexperienced cook. The recipes are very versatile. In many cases, you can change the meat or fish suggested, to make an equally tasty dish.

When shopping, see which are the best foods available. Many of the most highly regarded chefs choose their menus after seeing for themselves which the freshest foods are at the market!

If it is more convenient to prepare, for instance, Day 5's recipes on Day 3, then do so, as long as within the week you are eating a balance of meat, fish, vegetables, fruit and grains. Some people prefer to eat their main meal at lunchtime and their light meal in the evening, whereas for others it is more practical to do the reverse. Therefore, adapt the diet according to your lifestyle, to your personal diata.

The diet is laid out in such a way that, starting on a Monday, the slightly more elaborate meals are at the weekend. If you wish to start on another day, by all means do so; simply change the order within the week if you so wish.

Bearing in mind that many people eat lunch at work, most of the light meal dishes can be taken to work either in a food container or, for a more filling lunch, pocketed in some pita bread.

Add more spices, herbs or garlic if this is to your taste. Adapt some of your own favorite recipes to low fat versions by using methods suggested in these recipes, such as cooking onions in water or in chopped tomatoes instead of frying them.

A meal should be an occasion enjoyed by all. Too many people nowadays seem to eat while watching television, hardly noticing what or how much they are eating. How much nicer for a family or friends or even just oneself to sit at a table set for a meal!

If one is entertaining friends or business colleagues, it is nice to offer three courses, but this does not have to be the case every day. When eating on your own or with the family, serve a variety of crudités (raw vegetables) with a squeeze of fresh lemon juice or with a little reduced calorie mayonnaise seasoned with herbs as a dip. Thin strips of carrot, celery, cucumber and bell pepper, cauliflower florets and Belgian endive leaves are all excellent foods, taste good and look appetizing. Generally, eat fresh fruit or low-fat or fat-free yogurt as a dessert. Take advantage of the enormous variety of fruit available. Whatever the circumstances, always present the food in an attractive way.

BREAKFAST

After approximately ten hours of fasting, the body needs a good source of energy for the demands of the day to come. Many people make do with a cup of coffee which, although it may taste good, does little to support you until lunchtime. And it may tempt you into a mid-morning snack of chocolate cookies or worse.

People who skip breakfast work less efficiently than people who have taken the trouble to provide themselves with fuel for the morning. Other people, however, have a long tradition of breakfasting wholeheartedly, but perhaps in a way that is not wholesome for the heart.

Breakfast cereals—hot or cold—are an excellent source of energy. They are generally high in complex carbohydrates as well as fiber. Read labels, though, to make sure your choices are low in fat, salt and sugar. As a change and to provide more nourishment, try topping them with yogurt and/or fresh fruit. Try making your own muesli rather than buying well-known brands.

Eggs are a good source of protein but they should be cooked without using fat and eaten in moderation, especially by those watching their cholesterol. Poach, boil or scramble the eggs, or make into an omelette in a non-stick pan with a bit of low fat margarine or cooking spray. Chop a little low-fat cheese, tomato or mushroom into a scrambled egg or an omelette as a variation. Add small pieces of smoked salmon for a delicious breakfast!

Eating fruit is a very refreshing start to the day. Chop and mix together two or three kinds of fresh fruit. Squeeze a little fresh orange juice over the fruit—you can almost taste the energy!

Freshly juiced vegetables or fruit provide an excellent meal-in-a-glass. Carrot juice contains many vitamins, including vitamin A, and is the ideal mixer for other vegetable juices. It can easily be mixed with orange or apple juice, if preferred. Experiment with different juices and combinations.

With a little time and imagination, there is no end to the low fat, high fiber energy breakfasts you can make for yourself.

BREAKFAST RECIPES

Muesli

2 tablespoons oats
2 teaspoons bran
1 teaspoon split almonds
1 teaspoon pumpkin seeds
1 teaspoon sesame seeds
1 apple, cut into small pieces or grated
2 teaspoons raisins
skim milk
non-fat plain yogurt

Soak the oats and bran in skim milk overnight. Add all other ingredients and mix thoroughly. Top with non-fat plain yogurt.

Fruit Yogurt

2 cups non-fat plain yogurt
1 nectarine
½ cup raspberries
2 teaspoons clear honey

Put the yogurt into bowls. Arrange the raspberries on top in the middle. Cut each nectarine half into 4 slices and arrange around the raspberries. Drizzle the honey over the fruit.

LUNCH AND DINNER RECIPES

Please note:
All recipes are for two people. Simple halve or multiply quantities as required.

DAY 1

LUNCH **Greek Salad**

crispy lettuce leaves, such as iceberg
1 large tomato, cut into wedges
piece of cucumber, cut into wedges
raw onion rings (soaked in cold water for half an hour if possible)
3 ounces feta cheese
8 black olives
2 lemon wedges
lemon juice
freshly ground black pepper

Arrange salad, squeeze some lemon juice over and add freshly ground pepper. Garnish with the lemon wedges and serve with one piece of pita bread or one slice whole grain bread per person.

DINNER   ## Salmon Risotto

> 6 ounces boneless fresh salmon
>   or 1 8-ounce can of salmon
> 1 medium onion, chopped
> 1 small can of sweet corn, drained
> ½ cup frozen peas
> 1½ cups fish stock
> 1 cup white wine and water, mixed
> 2 teaspoons light soy sauce
> freshly ground black pepper and salt
> ½ cup Italian rice, uncooked
> 1 teaspoon vegetable oil
> 2 lime wedges

If using fresh salmon, poach the salmon in the white wine and water for 5 minutes. Remove the salmon. Cook the onion and peas gently in the cooking liquid for 10 minutes, then put with the salmon, reserving the cooking juices. Add the fish stock to the juices and keep warm. In another pan, warm the vegetable oil. Add the rice and, stirring continuously, cook for 2-3 minutes. Add ¾ cup of the stock to the rice and simmer, stirring occasionally, until the liquid is absorbed. Add another ¾ cup of the stock, repeating the process. Finally, add the light soy sauce and the salt and pepper. If the rice is still not cooked, add a small amount of water. Stir in the sweet corn, peas and onion and finally, for a few moments, the salmon. Garnish with the lime wedges.

DAY 2

LUNCH   ## Chicken Dijon Sandwich

> 2 teaspoon Dijon mustard
> 2 tablespoons low-fat cottage cheese
> 1 teaspoon thyme
> 2 slices whole grain bread
> 6 ounces chicken or turkey breast, thinly sliced
> salt and pepper

In a bowl, mix the dijon mustard, cottage cheese and thyme. Spread evenly over bread. Place slices of chicken or turkey on top and add salt and pepper to taste. Serve with fresh fruit.

DINNER   ## Eggplant à l'Italienne

> 1 large eggplant
> 1 medium onion
> 1 8-ounce can of tomatoes
> 1 medium red bell pepper
> 1 cup (¼ pound) mushrooms
> 4 ounces mozzarella cheese
> 2 teaspoons grated Parmesan cheese
> 2 teaspoons chopped fresh basil
>   or 1 teaspoon dried mixed herbs
> 1 clove garlic, chopped
> freshly ground black pepper and salt

Slice the eggplant into 1/3" thick rings and chop the onion. Cook together in boiling, salted water for 10 minutes. Drain and arrange in an ovenproof dish. Chop the red pepper and mushrooms and arrange on the eggplant. Pour the tomatoes over the vegetables. Add the garlic, herbs, salt and pepper. Slice the mozzarella cheese fairly thinly and arrange on the vegetables. Sprinkle the Parmesan cheese over the top. Bake in a preheated oven at 400° for 30 minutes. Put under a hot broiler for a few moments until golden. Serve with a green salad.

DAY 3

LUNCH ### Strawberry and Cream Cheese Sandwich

12 large strawberries
4 tablespoons whipped low-fat cream cheese
4 slices whole grain bread

Hull strawberries and slice. Spread cream cheese over bread. Arrange strawberry halves over cream cheese.

DINNER ## Spaghetti Alle Vongole

1 can baby clams
1 medium onion, chopped
½ cup frozen peas
1 cup (¼ pound) mushrooms, sliced
1 16-ounce can chopped tomatoes
1 clove garlic, chopped
1 teaspoon chopped fresh parsley
  or ½ teaspoon dried mixed herbs
1 teaspoon tomato paste
¼ cup white wine or water
freshly ground black pepper and salt
4 ounces spaghetti (whole wheat)
2 lemon wedges

Cook the spaghetti as directed. Simmer the onion, garlic and peas in the tomatoes for 10 minutes. Add the mushrooms, herbs, tomato paste, wine or water, and salt and pepper. Finally add the clams. Cook until clams are heated through. Serve the spaghetti with the clam sauce poured over. Garnish with the lemon wedges.

DAY 4

LUNCH   ## Watercress and Kiwifruit Salad

> *watercress, or dark green, leafy lettuce*
> *2 kiwifruit, peeled and cut into pieces*
> *one small cucumber, cut into small pieces*
> *6 radishes, sliced*
> *1 teaspoon reduced-fat or non-fat mayonnaise*
> *2 teaspoons non-fat plain yogurt*
> *6 cashew nuts, chopped*
> *freshly ground black pepper*

Mix salad ingredients together. Combine mayonnaise and yogurt and mix with salad. Garnish with the chopped cashews and add some freshly ground black pepper. Serve with crusty brown bread.

DINNER   ## Frittata

> *1 medium onion, chopped*
> *1 red bell pepper, chopped*
> *2 medium potatoes, peeled, cut into ⅓" slices and*
>   *boiled*
> *½ teaspoon dried mixed herbs*
> *1 teaspoon vegetable oil*
> *3 eggs*
> *freshly ground black pepper and salt*

91

Cook the onion and red pepper in the vegetable oil in a non-stick frying pan. Add the cooked potato slices and the herbs. Whisk the eggs with a little water and some salt and pepper and pour over the vegetables. Cook until the frittata is set. Serve with a green salad.

DAY 5

LUNCH   ## Stuffed Bell Peppers

> *1 medium green bell pepper,*
> *cut in half lengthwise and de-seeded*
> *1 medium red bell pepper*
> *cut in half lengthwise and de-seeded*
> *1 medium onion, chopped*
> *1 clove garlic, chopped*
> *½ cup cooked brown rice*
> *1 8-ounce can of tomatoes*
> *1 teaspoon chopped fresh rosemary*
> *or ½ teaspoon dried mixed herbs*
> *freshly ground black pepper*

Simmer the onion and garlic in the tomatoes, herbs and black pepper. Add a little water if necessary. Remove the vegetables from the liquid and mix with the cooked rice. Arrange the rice and vegetable mixture in the pepper halves. Put them in an oven-proof dish. Increase the cooking liquid with water so it makes 1¼ cups and pour it over the peppers. Cover the dish and bake in a pre-heated oven at 375°, for 30 minutes.

DINNER ## Royal Indian Chicken

brown rice, 1 cup cooked
2 skinless, boneless chicken breasts, approx.
 5 ounces each
1 medium onion
1 cup (¼ pound) mushrooms, chopped
1 tablespoon finely chopped almonds
¾ cup non-fat plain yogurt
2 teaspoons curry powder
½ teaspoon hot chili powder
2 teaspoons lemon juice
1 cup water
freshly ground black pepper and salt
2 tablespoons toasted almonds

Cut the chicken into bite-size pieces and chop the onion. Poach gently in the water for 20 minutes. Add all other ingredients except the yogurt and toasted almonds. Stir carefully and cook for 10 more minutes. Reduce liquid if necessary. Add the yogurt. Garnish the chicken with toasted almonds. Serve with brown rice.

DAY 6

LUNCH ## Baked Potato with Kidney Beans

2 large baking potatoes
1 16-ounce can red kidney beans
2 teaspoons tomato paste
chili sauce to taste
lemon juice

Bake the potatoes until done, about 1 hour, or microwave until done, approx. 8-12 minutes. Heat the red kidney beans in the mixture of tomato paste, chili sauce and lemon juice, adding a little water if necessary. Open the potatoes lengthways and pile the kidney beans on top.

DINNER **Fish Pilaki**

6 ounces cod or other skinless white fish fillets
1 small onion, chopped
1 clove garlic, chopped
small bunch celery leaves, chopped
6 ounces tomatoes, skinned and chopped
1 tablespoon lemon juice
1 tablespoon chopped fresh parsley
freshly ground black pepper and salt
¾ cup fish stock
4 green olives, chopped

Simmer the onion, garlic, celery leaves and tomatoes in the fish stock for 10 minutes, then add the fish. Cook gently for 10 more minutes, then break the fish into bite-size pieces. Reduce the liquid. Stir in the lemon juice and parsley and add salt and pepper to taste. Garnish with chopped green olives. Serve with a tomato and onion salad and a slice of whole grain bread.

DAY 7

LUNCH ## Salade Niçoise

1 6⅛-ounce can water-packed tuna fish, drained
1 can anchovies, soaked in milk to reduce saltiness
1 hard-boiled egg, quartered
8 green or black olives
watercress or any other salad leaf
1 large tomato, diced
1 small green bell pepper, diced
1 small onion, chopped finely
1 clove garlic, chopped finely
2 teaspoons lemon juice
1 teaspoon olive oil
freshly ground black pepper

Combine all salad ingredients with the flaked tuna. Toss, in the dressing of lemon juice and olive oil. Decorate with the anchovies, olives and quarters of hard-boiled egg and finally grind some black pepper over the salad.

DINNER ## Turkey Provençal

skinless, boneless turkey breast, approx. ¾ pound
1 8-ounce can of tomatoes
1 medium onion, chopped
2 medium zucchini, sliced
1 cup (¼ pound) mushrooms, chopped
1 medium green or red bell pepper, chopped
2 ounces black olives
1 clove garlic
1 bouquet garni
   or ½ teaspoon dried mixed herbs
freshly ground black pepper and salt

Put the turkey, tomatoes, onion and zucchini into a pan with the garlic and herbs. Cook over a moderate heat for about 25 minutes. Add other vegetables and seasoning and cook for a further 10 minutes. Serve with a green salad.

DAY 8

LUNCH ## Apple Cheddar Melt

1 medium apple
4 ounces low-fat cheddar cheese
2 teaspoons reduced-fat or fat-free mayonnaise
4 thin slices pumpernickel or other dark bread

Core apple and cut into thin slices. Do not peel. Cut cheese into thin slices. Spread a bit of mayonnaise on each slice of bread. Arrange the apple slices over each slice of bread and top with cheese. Place the Apple Cheddar Melts one at a time on a paper towel on a microwavable plate and cook on medium power 1 minute, or until cheese melts. Don't overcook, as the bread will get hard.

These can also be heated under the broiler. Place under broiler until cheese melts.

DINNER   ## Mushrooms à la Grecque

3 cups (³⁄₄ pound) fresh mushrooms, chopped
1 medium onion, chopped
1 clove garlic, chopped
2 medium tomatoes, chopped
  or 1 8-ounce can of tomatoes
¹⁄₄ cup water (unless using canned tomatoes)
1 green bell pepper, chopped
1 teaspoon chopped fresh parsley
  or ¹⁄₂ teaspoon dried mixed herbs
1 bay leaf
freshly ground black pepper and salt
4 green olives, chopped

Cook the onion, garlic and tomatoes in the water for 10 minutes. Add all other ingredients except the olives and cook for a further 5 minutes. Garnish with the chopped green olives and serve with brown rice and a green salad.

DAY 9

LUNCH   ## Insalata Caprese

1 large ripe tomato, sliced
4 ounces sliced, part skim-milk mozzarella cheese
4 teaspoons fresh basil, shredded, or ¹⁄₂ teaspoon dried
2 teaspoons olive oil
2 slices Italian bread

Arrange tomato slices on plate. Top with mozzarella, and then the basil. Drizzle the olive oil over the salad. Serve with one slice of Italian bread per person.

DINNER ## Penne with Ham

> 4 ounces penne, or other pasta
> 4 ounces cooked ham, cut into strips
> ½ cup frozen peas
> 1 medium onion, chopped
> 1 clove garlic, chopped
> 2 medium zucchini, cut into small pieces
> 1 cup (¼ pound) mushrooms, chopped
> 1 teaspoon chopped fresh thyme
>   or ½ teaspoon dried mixed herbs
> dash Tabasco or chili sauce to taste
> 1 8-ounce can of tomatoes
> freshly ground black pepper and salt

Cook the pasta as directed. Cook all other ingredients, except the ham, in the tomatoes, with a little added water if necessary, for 10 minutes. Add the ham and cook until ham is heated through. Stir the pasta into the sauce. Serve with a bit of grated Parmesan cheese if desired and a green salad.

DAY 10

LUNCH ## Sweet Corn and Red Bell Pepper Salad

> 1 large can sweet corn
> 1 medium red bell pepper
> 1 small onion
> 2 teaspoons reduced-fat or fat-free mayonnaise
> cayenne pepper

Cut the red pepper into small pieces and grate the onion. Mix together with the sweet corn and mayonnaise. Add a pinch of cayenne pepper. Serve with a slice of whole grain bread.

DINNER ## Ginger Orange Fish

brown rice, 1 cup cooked
8 ounces firm white fish fillets, such as cod or monkfish
juice of 2 oranges
½" piece ginger root, peeled and shredded
freshly ground black pepper

Place the fish in a parcel of foil with the orange juice, ginger and black pepper. Bake in a preheated oven, at 400°, for 25 minutes. Serve with brown rice and a Belgian endive and orange salad.

DAY 11

LUNCH ## Open Faced Waldorf Sandwich

2 sticks celery
1 red apple
1 green apple
2 teaspoons chopped walnuts
1 small onion
1 tablespoon non-fat plain yogurt
lemon juice
freshly ground black pepper

Cut the celery and apples into small pieces and grate the onion. Mix together all ingredients and pile onto whole grain bread, one slice for each serving.

DINNER   ## Broccoli Mornay

1 pound broccoli, cut lengthwise
1 medium onion, chopped
2 eggs, hard-boiled
6 ounces cheese (low-fat, if possible), grated
1¼ cups skim milk
2 tablespoons cornstarch, mixed with a little water
freshly ground black pepper and salt

Cook the broccoli and onion in a steamer for 10 minutes. Arrange in an ovenproof dish and put slices of hard-boiled egg on top. Add salt and pepper. Make a white sauce with the milk and cornstarch and add most of the grated cheese. Pour the sauce over the broccoli and egg. Scatter the remaining grated cheese over the top. Bake in a pre-heated oven, at 375°, for 15 minutes, then brown under the broiler. Serve with baked potatoes and a green salad.

DAY 12

LUNCH   ## Pasta Salad Primavera

2 ounces pasta, cooked
2 medium tomatoes, diced
1 small cucumber, diced
8 capers
1 teaspoon reduced-fat or fat-free mayonnaise
2 teaspoons non-fat plain yogurt
dash of soy sauce
freshly ground black pepper
2 lemon wedges

Combine all ingredients and chill if desired. Arrange on a plate and garnish with the lemon wedges.

DINNER   ## Chinese Pork Tenderloin with Shrimp

> *1 cup brown rice, cooked*
> *4 ounces pork tenderloin*
> *4 ounces cooked shrimp*
> *2 sticks of celery, chopped*
> *1 medium onion, chopped*
> *1 clove garlic, chopped*
> *1 cup (¼ pound) mushrooms, chopped*
> *1 teaspoon soy sauce*
> *1 teaspoon teriyaki sauce (optional)*
> *¾ cup water, or wine and water, mixed*
> *1 teaspoon lemon juice*
> *freshly ground black pepper and salt*

Prepare brown rice. Bake the pork tenderloin with the lemon juice in foil for 25 minutes in a preheated oven, at 400°. When cooked, shred the meat, reserving any juices. Meanwhile, in a wok or a large pan, gently poach the chopped celery, onion and garlic in the wine/water for 5 minutes. Add the chopped mushrooms and cook for 5 more minutes. Stir in the soy and teriyaki sauce, then add the pork, with any remaining juices, and the shrimp. Add salt and pepper. Serve with brown rice.

DAY 13

LUNCH   ## Baked Potato with Cottage Cheese and Kiwifruit

> *2 large baking potatoes*
> *8 ounces low-fat cottage cheese*
> *2 kiwifruit, peeled*

Bake the potatoes, then open them lengthways. Pile the cottage cheese onto the potatoes and arrange slices of kiwifruit on top.

DINNER ## Light Fettuccine Alfredo

4 ounces fettuccine
2 teaspoon margarine
1 tablespoon light cream
2 tablespoons plain, low-fat yogurt
3 tablespoons Parmesan cheese, freshly grated
  if available
salt and pepper

Cook fettuccine as directed. Drain, reserving three tablespoons of the cooking water. Place fettuccine in serving bowl and toss with margarine, reserved cooking water, cream, yogurt, Parmesan cheese, and salt and pepper to taste. Serve with a green salad and one slice Italian bread for each serving.

Note: There are many flavored pastas available—spinach, basil, and tomato, to name a few—and any of them can be substituted for the regular fettuccine to make a delicious variation on this dish.

DAY 14

LUNCH ## Spinach and Tuna Salad

1 6¼-ounce can water-packed tuna fish, drained
  raw spinach leaves, washed and shredded
1 medium tomato, chopped
2 teaspoons reduced fat or fat-free mayonnaise
  freshly ground black pepper
2 lime wedges

Flake the tuna. Mix together with the tomato and mayonnaise. Serve on individual plates on the shredded spinach leaves, garnished with the lime wedges. Grind some black pepper over the salad. Serve with crusty brown bread.

DINNER **Chicken Lombattini**

*2 skinless, boneless chicken breasts, approx. 5 ounces
  each
1 cup (¼ pound) mushrooms, sliced
1 teaspoon lemon juice
dash Tabasco or chili sauce
1/3 cup white wine
1 teaspoon chopped fresh basil
  or ½ teaspoon dried mixed herbs
2 teaspoons olive oil
freshly ground black pepper and salt
2 lemon wedges*

Cook the chicken gently in the olive oil for about 8 minutes. Add the mushrooms. Add wine, lemon juice and Tabasco or chili sauce. Add herbs, salt and pepper. Garnish with the lemon wedges. Serve with boiled new potatoes and green beans.

DAY 15

LUNCH **Lentil and Tomato Salad**

*½ cup lentils, soaked and cooked as directed
2 medium tomatoes, sliced
1 small onion, grated or cut into small pieces
½ teaspoon mustard
lemon juice
freshly ground black pepper*

Mix together the lentils, onion and mustard. Put on a plate and arrange the tomato on top. Squeeze some lemon juice and grind some black pepper onto the salad.

DINNER ## Tagliatelle With Shrimp

4 ounces tagliatelle, or other pasta
2 tablespoons olive oil
1 medium onion, chopped
1 clove garlic, chopped
6 ounces shrimp, shelled and deveined
1 cup (¼ pound) mushrooms, chopped
½ cup sweet corn
1 teaspoon chopped fresh dill
  or ½ teaspoon dried mixed herbs
2 teaspoons light soy sauce
freshly ground black pepper and salt

Cook the pasta as directed. Cook the onion and garlic in a little water for 10 minutes. Sauté the shrimp, mushrooms, sweet corn and dill or mixed herbs and cook for 4-5 minutes. Add the onion and garlic mixture and reduce liquid if necessary. Add the light soy sauce and pepper and salt to taste. Arrange the pasta on a serving dish and pour the sauce over it. Serve with a green bell pepper and cucumber salad.

DAY 16

LUNCH ## Zucchini and Mushrooms With Rice

2 medium zucchini, sliced
1 cup (¼ pound) mushrooms, chopped
1 small onion, chopped
½ cup cooked brown rice
1 teaspoon chopped fresh parsley
  or ½ teaspoon dried mixed herbs
soy sauce
lemon juice
freshly ground black pepper and salt
black olives

Gently simmer the zucchini, mushrooms, onion and herbs in water for 10 minutes. Reduce the liquid. Mix vegetables with the rice, soy sauce, lemon juice and pepper and salt. Garnish with black olives.

DINNER · **Tarragon Chicken**

3 tablespoons dry white wine
2 teaspoons olive oil
½ teaspoon dried tarragon
¼ teaspoon salt
¼ teaspoon pepper
2 skinned chicken breasts, approx. 8 ounces each

In a bowl, mix wine, olive oil, tarragon, salt and pepper. Add chicken and marinate at room temperature for 30-45 minutes, turning chicken over once or twice. After chicken is marinated, preheat broiler. Remove chicken from marinade, saving remaining marinade for basting. Place chicken, bone side up, about 6 inches from heat. Broil for 10 minutes. Turn over and baste with remaining marinade and broil 10-15 minutes more, or until done. Serve with boiled new potatoes seasoned with mixed herbs—2 medium or 3 small for each person—and a green salad.

DAY 17

LUNCH · **Crab and Dill Omelette**

5 ounces fresh or canned crabmeat, or imitation
  crabmeat
2 eggs plus 2 egg whites
1 teaspoon chopped fresh dill
2 small sprigs of dill for garnish
freshly ground black pepper and salt
radicchio or other salad leaves
2 lime wedges

Whisk the eggs with a little water, adding pepper and salt and the chopped dill. Stir into this mixture half of the crabmeat. Using a non-stick omelette pan, adding a little oil or cooking spray, cook the omelette. At the last moment, add the rest of the crabmeat and fold the omelette over. Cut in half and put a sprig of dill on each half. Serve on individual plates, each garnished with radicchio leaves and a lime wedge.

DINNER   ## Mushroom Risotto

*3 cups mushrooms, chopped (¼ pound each of
    different types if possible)*
1 medium onion, chopped
1 clove garlic, chopped
½ cup frozen peas
½ cup cooked or canned Garbanzo beans
1½ cups vegetable stock
1 cup white wine and water, mixed
*1 teaspoon chopped fresh thyme
    or ½ teaspoon dried mixed herbs*
½ cup Italian rice
1 teaspoon vegetable oil
freshly ground black pepper and salt
2 lemon wedges

Gently cook the mushrooms, peas, onion and garlic in the vegetable stock and herbs for 5 minutes. Remove the vegetables. Add the wine and water to the cooking liquid. In another pan, warm the vegetable oil. Add the rice and, stirring continuously, cook for 2-3 minutes. Add ¾ cup of the cooking liquid to the rice and simmer, stirring occasionally, until the liquid is absorbed. Add a further ¾ cup of the liquid, repeating the process. Finally, add the rest of the liquid and the pepper and salt. If the rice is still not cooked, add some more water. Stir in all the vegetables and garnish with the lemon wedges. Serve with a tomato and cucumber salad.

DAY 18

LUNCH   ## Tabouli

½ cup bulgur (cracked wheat)
1 large tomato, diced
1 medium cucumber, diced
1 small onion, grated
1 tablespoon chopped fresh mint
juice of 1 large lemon
1 teaspoon olive oil
freshly ground black pepper and salt
2 lemon wedges

Soak the bulgar in lots of cold water for 15 minutes, then rinse and drain, squeezing the water out. Put in a bowl with the lemon juice and the pepper and salt. Leave for a few minutes. Add the olive oil, mint and salad ingredients and mix thoroughly. Garnish with the lemon wedges.

DINNER   ## Fish Provençal

8 ounces skinless white fish fillets such as
*   cod or monkfish*
1 8-ounce can of tomatoes
1 medium onion, finely chopped
1 teaspoon chopped fresh parsley
*   or ½ teaspoon dried mixed herbs*
1 clove garlic, chopped
1 teaspoon lemon juice
2 lemon wedges
freshly ground black pepper and salt

Place the fish in an ovenproof serving dish. Add all other ingredients except the lemon wedges. Cover with foil and bake for 15 minutes in a preheated oven, at 400°. Remove the foil and bake for 5 more minutes. Garnish with the lemon wedges. Serve with baked potatoes and a green salad.

DAY 19

LUNCH **Belgian Endive, Orange and Cucumber Salad**

1 head Belgian endive, cut into rings
1 orange, peeled and sliced
one small cucumber, sliced
2 teaspoons non-fat plain yogurt
orange juice
freshly ground black pepper

Combine salad ingredients with the yogurt and pepper. Squeeze some fresh orange juice over the salad and serve with a slice of whole grain bread.

DINNER **Turkey Jambalaya**

2 skinless, boneless turkey breasts, approx. ½ pound,
   cut into small pieces
2 teaspoons lemon juice
1 medium onion, chopped
1 cup skinned and chopped fresh tomato
   or 1 8-ounce can of tomatoes
1 8-ounce can red kidney beans, drained
2 stalks celery, chopped
1 teaspoon chopped fresh basil
1 teaspoon chopped fresh parsley
1 bay leaf
2 chopped green onions
½ cup brown rice, uncooked
Tabasco or chili sauce (optional)
salt and cayenne pepper
2 lime wedges

Put the turkey with the lemon juice into an ovenproof dish. Cover with foil and bake for 25 minutes in a preheated oven, at 400°. Meanwhile cook the rice and in another pan, cook the onion and celery with the tomatoes and ¾ cup water. (If using canned tomatoes omit the water.) Add the basil, parsley and bay leaf, salt and cayenne pepper. Stir the rice into the tomato mixture, adding Tabasco or chili sauce to taste, if desired. Add the beans, pour over the turkey, mix well and continue to cook, covered, in the oven for another 10 minutes or until the meat is cooked. Garnish with chopped green onions and the lime wedges.

DAY 20

LUNCH ## Tuna and Red Kidney Bean Salad

1 8-ounce can of water-packed tuna fish, drained
1 8-ounce can of red kidney beans, drained
1 small onion, finely chopped
lemon juice
freshly ground black pepper
4 Belgian endive leaves, or other salad leaves

Mix the tuna, red kidney beans and onion together. Squeeze some lemon juice over and add freshly ground pepper. Garnish with endive leaves cut into rings. Serve with a slice of whole grain bread.

DINNER   ## Mediterranean Vegetables

1 large zucchini
1 large green bell pepper
1 large tomato
1 small onion
1 clove garlic
½ cup cooked brown rice
1 teaspoon soy sauce
1 teaspoon tomato paste
¾ cup white wine and water, mixed
2 teaspoons chopped fresh basil
*   or 1 teaspoon dried mixed herbs*
freshly ground black pepper and salt
lightly toasted pine nuts or flaked almonds

Cut the zucchini in half lengthways and scoop out inner flesh. Cut the bell pepper in half lengthways and remove seeds and stem. Cut the tomato in half and scoop out flesh. Cook the chopped onion, garlic, zucchini flesh and tomato flesh in the wine and water mixed with the soy sauce and tomato paste. When cooked, drain and reserve the liquid. Add the rice, herbs, salt and pepper to the onion mixture. Arrange in the vegetable shells. Put them in an ovenproof dish and add the cooking liquid, adding some water if necessary. Cover with foil and bake for 30 minutes in a preheated oven, at 400°. Garnish with the nuts. Serve with a slice of whole grain bread.

DAY 21

LUNCH ## Gazpacho

> 1 pound tomatoes, skinned
>   or 1 16-ounce can of chopped tomatoes
> 2 medium zucchini
> 1 small onion
> 1/4 cucumber
> 1/2 green bell pepper
> 1 clove garlic
> 2 teaspoons chopped fresh basil
>   or 1 teaspoon dried mixed herbs
> 1 1/4 cups chicken stock
> 3/4 cup water or white wine mixed with water
> freshly ground black pepper and salt

Chop vegetables; then blend all ingredients in a food processor or blender. Chill for at least 2 hours. (If short of time, add a few ice cubes). Serve separate small bowls of chopped cucumber, onion, red and green bell pepper for garnish. Serve with one slice whole grain bread per person.

DINNER ## Venetian Shrimp

> 6 ounces cooked shrimp
> 2 medium tomatoes, chopped
> 1 small onion, cut into small pieces
> 1 clove garlic, chopped
> 1 teaspoon chopped fresh parsley
>   or 1/2 teaspoon dried mixed herbs
> 5/8 cup white wine and water mixed
> 2 teaspoons light soy sauce
> freshly ground black pepper

111

Gently cook the tomatoes, onion and garlic in the white wine and water. Add the herbs, light soy sauce and black pepper. Reduce the liquid if necessary. Add the shrimp until heated through. Serve with herbed brown rice.

DAY 22

LUNCH   **Curried Chicken and Orange Salad**

> 1 cup cooked chicken breast cut into ½-inch cubes
> ½ cup diced celery
> 1 orange, peeled and sectioned
> ½ teaspoon curry powder
> 2 teaspoons diced onion
> ¼ cup reduced-fat or fat-free mayonnaise
> salt and pepper, to taste

In a bowl, mix all of the ingredients until chicken is evenly coated. Serve on a bed of lettuce.

DINNER   **Celery Provençal**

> 1 cup brown rice, cooked
> 1 head of celery
> 1 16-ounce can of tomatoes
> 1 medium onion, chopped
> 1 clove garlic, chopped
> 1 cup (¼ pound) mushrooms, chopped
> 1 red bell pepper, chopped
> 1 teaspoon chopped fresh parsley
>   or ½ teaspoon dried mixed herbs
> freshly ground black pepper and salt

Trim the celery and cut into large pieces. Cook all ingredients except the mushrooms and bell pepper over a medium heat for 20 minutes, adding some water if necessary. Add the mushrooms and pepper and cook for 10 more minutes. Serve with brown rice.

DAY 23

LUNCH ## Huevos Rancheros

¼ cup salsa
2 tablespoons water
2 eggs plus 2 egg whites
1 green onion, chopped
2 teaspoons reduced-fat sour cream

Mix salsa and water and cook over medium heat until heated through. In a non-stick pan sprayed with cooking spray, scramble the eggs and egg whites with the green onions. To serve, ladle the salsa evenly onto two plates and place the scrambled eggs on top. Garnish with a dollop of sour cream and chopped green onion. Serve with one tortilla or one slice whole grain bread per person.

DINNER ## Saumon Aux Épinards

2 5-ounce fillets of fresh salmon
10–12 large spinach leaves
2 lime wedges

Blanch the spinach leaves in boiling water for about 30 seconds, then dry with a paper towel. Wrap 5–6 leaves around each piece of salmon. Steam in a vegetable steamer over simmering water for 5 minutes. Garnish with the lime wedges and serve with boiled new potatoes and green beans.

DAY 24

LUNCH **Open-Faced Avocado and Swiss Sandwich**

1 tablespoon reduced-fat or fat-free mayonnaise
1 tablespoon Dijon mustard
½ cup sprouts
4 slices thinly sliced pumpernickel or other dark bread
2 1-ounce slices of Swiss cheese, cut into 2-inch strips
½ small avocado, cut into thin slices

Mix mayonnaise and mustard together. Spread over the slices of bread. Evenly distribute the sprouts on the bread. Place cheese slices on sprouts; then add avocado slices.

DINNER **Lemon Chicken Breasts**

Juice from ½ fresh lemon
½ teaspoon grated lemon zest
1 tablespoon vegetable oil
salt and pepper
2 skinless chicken breasts, approx. 8 ounces each
2 lemon wedges

In a bowl, mix lemon juice, lemon zest, oil, salt and pepper. Add chicken breasts and turn over to coat with marinade. Marinate at room temperature for 30-45 minutes, turning chicken over once or twice. After chicken is marinated, preheat broiler. Remove chicken from marinade, reserving remaining marinade for basting. Place chicken, bone side up, about 6 inches from heat. Broil for 10 minutes. Turn over and baste with remaining marinade and broil 10-15 minutes more, or until done. Serve with herbed rice and a green salad.

DAY 25

LUNCH ## Mushroom Pizza Melt

¼ *cup tomato sauce*
2 *English muffins*
¼ *teaspoon oregano*
¼ *teaspoon basil*
4 *medium sized mushrooms, sliced*
¼ *cup part skim-milk mozzarella cheese*
1 *tablespoon grated Parmesan cheese*

Preheat broiler. Spread tomato sauce over the English muffin halves. Season with oregano and basil. Top each muffin with thinly sliced mushrooms. Sprinkle each muffin with mozzarella and Parmesan cheese. Place muffins on broiler, 6 inches from heat and broil until cheese is melted.

DINNER ## Tuna Tortiglioni

4 *ounces tortiglioni, or other pasta*
6 *ounces fresh tuna, grilled for 5 minutes, then flaked*
or 1 6¼-ounce can water-packed tuna, drained
1 *medium onion, chopped*
1 *clove garlic, chopped*
1 *cup (¼ pound) mushrooms, chopped*
2 *stalks celery, chopped*
1 *8-ounce can of tomatoes*
1 *bouquet garni*
or ½ teaspoon dried mixed herbs
½ *cup white wine and water mixed*
freshly ground black pepper and salt

Cook the pasta as directed. Cook the onion, garlic, mushrooms and celery in the tomatoes and wine/water with the bouquet garni or mixed herbs. Add the flaked tuna and pepper and salt, then mix with the pasta. Serve with a green salad.

DAY 26

LUNCH   ## Island Fruit Salad

1 cup pineapple chunks, fresh if available
1 banana, peeled and sliced
1 kiwi, peeled and sliced
1 cup low-fat cottage cheese
2 tablespoons low-fat plain yogurt

In a bowl, combine fruit. In another bowl, mix together the cottage cheese and the yogurt. Divide the fruit mixture into two bowls and top with the cottage cheese and yogurt.

DINNER   ## Baked Snapper Teriyaki

1 tablespoon soy sauce
½ clove garlic, finely chopped
½ teaspoon ginger root, finely chopped
¼ cup water
2 tablespoons dry white wine
2 red snapper fillets (or similar white fish),
    approx. 4 ounces each

Preheat oven to 450°. In a shallow ovenproof dish, mix soy sauce, garlic, ginger, water and white wine. Place snapper fillets in dish. Bake 10-12 minutes, basting 2 or 3 times with the sauce during the baking. Serve with brown rice and steamed broccoli and water chestnuts.

DAY 27

LUNCH   ## Lentil Soup with Cilantro

½ cup lentils
1 small whole onion
1 garlic clove, finely chopped
1 bay leaf
3 cups water
salt and ground pepper to taste
2 tablespoons chopped cilantro
2 tablespoons reduced fat sour cream for garnish

Combine the lentils, onion, garlic, bay leaf, and water in a large saucepan. Bring to a boil, reduce the heat, and simmer for 40 minutes. Remove from the heat. Discard the onion and bay leaf. Add salt and pepper to taste, stir in the cilantro, and serve, topping each bowl with a dollop of sour cream.

DINNER   ## Paella

2 small skinless boneless chicken breasts, approx.
  4 ounces each
4 ounces cooked shrimp
½ cup rice
1 medium onion
½ cup frozen peas
1 cup (¼ pound) mushrooms, chopped
1 medium green or red bell pepper, chopped
1 clove garlic
2 teaspoons chopped fresh parsley
  or 1 teaspoon dried mixed herbs
1 teaspoon lemon juice
freshly ground black pepper and salt
½ teaspoon turmeric powder
2 lemon wedges

117

A wok is ideal for making paella; otherwise use a large frying pan. Cook rice as directed in a medium pan, adding the turmeric to the water. Chop onion and chicken into small pieces and cook with the peas in water or, if desired, white wine with water, in the wok or frying pan for 15 minutes. Add the mushrooms, bell pepper, garlic and herbs. Add rice to the pan, and also fish sauce, lemon juice and salt and pepper to taste. Immediately prior to serving, add the shrimp and mix all ingredients. Garnish with the lemon wedges.

DAY 28

LUNCH   ## Zucchini and Mushroom Salad

2 medium zucchini, finely sliced
1 cup (¼ pound) mushrooms, finely sliced
2 teaspoons lemon juice
1 teaspoon olive oil
1 teaspoon chopped fresh parsley
    or ½ teaspoon dried mixed herbs
freshly ground black pepper

Combine all ingredients and if possible leave for 20 minutes for flavors to blend. Serve with a slice of whole grain bread.

DINNER   ## Mexican Beef

6 ounces lean steak
1 medium onion
1 clove garlic
1 green bell pepper
1 red bell pepper
1 cup (¼ pound) mushrooms
1 8-ounce can red kidney beans, drained
½ green chili, de-seeded - optional
1 teaspoon tomato paste
¾ cup water, or wine and water, mixed
chili sauce
2 teaspoons vegetable oil
freshly ground black pepper and salt

Poach the chopped onion and garlic in the wine/water for 5 minutes. Add the chopped, de-seeded peppers and chili and the sliced mushrooms, then cook for 5 more minutes. Remove the vegetables and keep warm. Reduce the juices and stir in the tomato paste, chili sauce and salt and pepper. Return the vegetables to the pan and keep warm, then add the red kidney beans. Meanwhile, cut the steak into slivers, ½″ wide by 1″, as thinly as possible—this is more easily done if the meat is put into the freezer about 30 minutes before being cut. Gently cook in the vegetable oil for 3-4 minutes. Stir the meat into the vegetables and serve immediately with brown rice and a green salad.

DAY 29

LUNCH **Pasta and Bell Pepper Salad**

2 ounces pasta, cooked
1 small red bell pepper, diced
1 small green bell pepper, diced
small bunch of grapes, halved and seeded
1 teaspoon reduced-fat or fat-free mayonnaise
2 teaspoons non-fat plain yogurt
freshly ground black pepper

Mix together the pasta, peppers, mayonnaise and yogurt. Garnish with the grapes and grind some black pepper over the salad.

DINNER **Sweet Corn Mornay**

2 corn cobs, corn sliced off
* or 1 large can sweet corn, drained*
2 eggs, hard-boiled and cut into pieces
½ cup non-fat plain yogurt
5 ounces cheese (low-fat, if possible), grated
freshly ground black pepper

Mix together the corn, egg and yogurt and put into an ovenproof dish. Sprinkle the grated cheese over the top and grind some black pepper onto the dish. Bake in a pre-heated oven, at 375° for 15 minutes. Brown under the broiler. Serve with a tomato and onion salad and a slice of whole grain bread.

DAY 30

LUNCH ## Shrimp and Rice Salad

4 ounces cooked shrimp
1/4 cup brown rice
1/4 cup frozen peas
1/2 teaspoon soy sauce
1 teaspoon lemon juice
1 teaspoon reduced-fat or fat-free mayonnaise
freshly ground black pepper and salt
2 sprigs of parsley

Cook the rice, and add the peas to the rice for the last few minutes. Chill. When the rice and peas are cold, mix in the shrimp. Gently stir in the other ingredients. Chill before serving. Garnish with the sprigs of parsley.

DINNER ## Chicken in Mint-and-Yogurt Marinade

2 skinless boneless chicken breasts, approx. 4 ounces
  each
1/3 cup non-fat plain yogurt
1 teaspoon chopped fresh mint
freshly ground black pepper
2 lemon wedges

Cut two slits into the top of each piece of chicken. Mix together the yogurt, mint and black pepper. Put the chicken into the marinade and leave for 15-30 minutes. Preheat broiler. Broil chicken, about 6 inches from heat, about 10 minutes on each side. Garnish with the lemon wedges and serve with a baked potato and green beans.

DAY	LUNCH
1	Greek Salad
2	Chicken Dijon Sandwich
3	Strawberry and Cream Cheese Sandwich
4	Watercress & Kiwifruit Salad
5	Stuffed Bell Peppers
6	Baked Potato with Kidney Beans
7	Salade Niçoise
8	Apple Cheddar Melt
9	Insalata Caprese
10	Sweet Corn & Red Bell Pepper Salad
11	Open-Faced Waldorf Salad
12	Pasta Salad Primavera
13	Baked Potato with Cottage Cheese & Kiwifruit
14	Spinach & Tuna Salad
15	Lentil & Tomato Salad
16	Zucchini & Mushrooms with Rice
17	Crab & Dill Omelette
18	Tabbouleh
19	Belgian Endive, Orange & Cucumber Salad
20	Tuna & Red Kidney Bean Salad
21	Gazpacho
22	Curried Chicken & Orange Salad
23	Huevos Rancheros
24	Open-Faced Avocado and Swiss Sandwich
25	Mushroom Pizza Melt
26	Island Fruit Salad
27	Lentil Soup with Cilantro
28	Zucchini & Mushroom Salad
29	Pasta & Pepper Salad
30	Shrimp & Rice Salad

DAY	DINNER
1	Salmon Risotto
2	Eggplant à l'Italienne
3	Spaghetti alle Vongole
4	Frittata
5	Royal Indian Chicken
6	Fish Pilaki
7	Turkey Provençal
8	Mushrooms à la Grecque
9	Penne with Ham
10	Ginger Orange Fish
11	Broccoli Mornay
12	Chinese Pork Tenderloin with Shrimp
13	Light Fettuccini Alfredo
14	Chicken Lombattini
15	Tagliatelle with Shrimp
16	Tarragon Chicken
17	Mushroom Risotto
18	Fish Provençal
19	Turkey Jambalaya
20	Mediterranean Vegetables
21	Venetian Shrimp
22	Celery Provençal
23	Saumon aux Épinards
24	Lemon Chicken Breasts
25	Tuna Tortiglioni
26	Baked Snapper Teriyaki
27	Paella
28	Mexican Beef
29	Sweet Corn Mornay
30	Chicken in Mint-and-Yogurt Marinade

SHOPPING LISTS

Life is often so busy that it is difficult always to have the necessary foods that you need on hand. The following lists are to help you stock up for The Walking Diet.

Pantry List

tomato paste
red kidney beans
canned water-packed tuna
canned clams
rice - brown
    white
    risotto
pasta - spaghetti - wholewheat
     tortiglioni
     penne
     tagliatelle
Tabasco or chili sauce
curry powder
olive oil
black peppercorns
ground almonds
pine nuts

canned chopped tomatoes
canned salmon
dried mixed herbs
bouquet garni
bulgar (cracked wheat)
sweet corn
olives
anchovies
eggs
artificial sweetener

vegetable oil
sea salt
split almonds
lentils
raisins
cereals

Refrigerator List

skim milk
reduced-fat or fat-free
  mayonnaise
cooked ham
feta cheese

low-fat spread or
  margarine
low-fat cottage cheese
non-fat plain yogurt
low-fat cheese

Freezer List

(many of these can be bought fresh, but if this is not possible, keep them in the freezer)

whole grain bread	pita bread
peas	fresh salmon
skinned boneless chicken breasts	pork tenderloin steak
skinned boneless turkey breasts	shrimp snow peas
ground beef	white fish

Market List

(to be bought as required)

watercress	lettuce, all varieties
Belgian endive	onions
zucchini	eggplant
celery	mushrooms
potatoes	spinach
bell peppers	sweet corn
apples	garlic
pears	oranges
raspberries	strawberries
lemons	grapes
figs	limes
melon - honeydew	mango
Cantaloupe	pineapple
watermelon	kiwifruit
bananas	tomatoes
nectarines	
herbs - parsley	
mint	
dill	
basil	

EATING OUT AND ENTERTAINING

Eating out won't be a problem when following The Walking Diet. Just follow these simple guidelines. Choose grilled fish or meat and ask for the accompanying vegetables to be served without butter, or have a salad, dressed simply with lemon juice rather than dressing. For dessert, select some fresh fruit. Most restaurants will be able to accommodate you.

If you are entertaining at home, use the dinner recipe from The Walking Diet for that day or choose another main meal recipe from your other favorite light dishes. Some of the lunch dishes could be used as a first course, such as Salade Niçoise, or Belgian Endive, Orange and Cucumber Salad.

·4·

THE
WALKER'S
WORKOUT

The wise for cure on exercise depend

JOHN DRYDEN

A warm-up routine is vital before brisk aerobic walking, because sudden vigorous activity can cause the heart to act abnormally. It can also lead to sprains, and torn muscles, tendons and ligaments.

Muscles work much better when relaxed, and it is much easier to find your stride and get into a good walking rhythm. The warm-up stretches in the quick routine that follows take only a few minutes, and should always be done before brisk walking. They relax the huge muscle on the front of the thigh (the quadriceps), the hamstring muscles at the back of the thigh, and the back of the calves and the Achilles tendons. They are followed by a further four warm-up stretches which you can do if you have the time. After these warm-up stretches, there are 20 stretches that provide you with flexibility and strength.

Walking is an excellent way of exercising the main muscle mass of the body (two-thirds of which is in the legs), and it will give you a good aerobic, cardiovascular work-out. But to achieve total body fitness you need to exercise all the main muscle groups in the body. The stretches for flexibility and strength will help you do this. A good workout several times a week will complement your aerobic walking routine and will help you build long term fitness.

The body is naturally designed to be flexible and to move and stretch easily. However, if you have been sedentary for some time and are not used to bending and stretching movements, then you are likely to be stiff and out of condition. You should approach the exercises for flexibility and strength with caution. You cannot expect to achieve all these positions as you start out, any more than you can expect to walk aerobically for 45 minutes when you first begin.

All the exercises are shown at full extension, so if you are unfit you should take particular care to build gradually towards the full exercise. Let the movements flow naturally; perform them slowly and smoothly and don't over-stretch. Ease into them gently.

The number of repetitions for each exercise and the length of time that poses are held are meant only as a guide—if necessary, reduce them to what you find comfortable. Similarly, as you progress week by week, you may wish to increase the intensity of the exercises to suit yourself. If you find any exercise too difficult to begin with, then leave it out until you gain the necessary strength and suppleness to approach it again. Take particular care with the strengthening exercises—push-ups, triceps and pectorals stretches. It is easy to overdo them. If necessary, begin with wall push-ups, graduating later to floor push-ups. If you listen to your body, you won't go wrong.

Like your aerobic walking, these exercises should leave you feeling relaxed and energized, not tired and aching. If

128

you feel tired and aching afterwards, then you are overdoing them. The key to performing them is to stretch slowly into them, letting the movements flow naturally.

If you have a specific back, neck or other problem that may prevent you from performing any of the stretching exercises in this chapter, then you should consult your family doctor before trying them—show him the exercises and ask his advice.

Cooling-down exercises after aerobic walking are just as important as warming-up exercises. Gradually reduce your pace as you come to the end of your walk. This will help you to avoid post-exercise stiffness and you will suffer from far less sore muscles. Then do the cool-down exercises, finishing with the total relaxation exercise.

THE WALKING DIET WARM-UP STRETCHES-QUICK ROUTINE

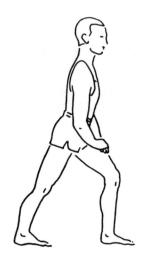

ACHILLES STRETCH
To stretch out the calves

Stand with your left foot forward. Bend it gently, keeping the right leg straight, heel on the ground. Both feet should be pointing forwards and you should support yourself by resting both hands on your left thigh. Hold for 10 seconds and repeat on the other side.

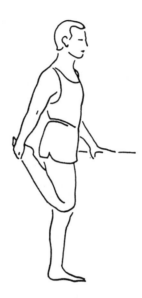

THIGH STRETCH
To stretch out the quadriceps down the front of the thigh

Stand on left leg, clasping right foot with left hand and using a chair for balance. Gently pull foot up, stretching the front of the right thigh. Keep you pelvis tucked forwards and knees close together. Hold for 15 seconds. Repeat on other side.

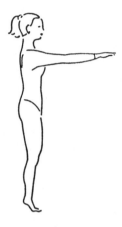

CALF RAISES
To strengthen the feet, ankles and calves

Stand with feet together, arms stretched out in front. (For balance, you might need to support yourself by resting your hands on the back of a chair.) Lift up on the balls of the feet. Hold for 5 seconds, then lower. Repeat 5 times.

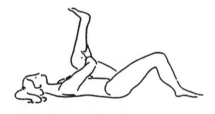

LYING HAMSTRING STRETCH
To improve suppleness

Lie on floor with knees bent and feet flat against ground. Draw left knee in towards chest, making sure you don't arch your back, and clasp with both hands just above knee. Slowly straighten leg until you feel a gentle stretch. Hold for 10-20 seconds. Repeat on other side.

132

FURTHER WARM-UP STRETCHES

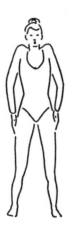

SHOULDER CIRCLES
To loosen and relax the neck, shoulders and back

Stand, arms at sides, with feet shoulder-width apart. Gently lift shoulders and move them backwards in a continuous rolling motion. Repeat 5 times, then repeat with a forward rolling motion.

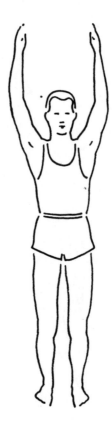

REACH FOR THE SKY
To increase circulation and activate and limber muscles

Stand with feet hip-width apart. Breathing in, bring hands up over your head so that you feel a mild stretching sensation lifting you upwards from your abdomen. Hold for the count of 5 and relax. Repeat 5 times.

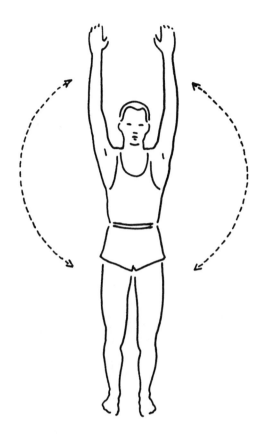

ARM CIRCLING
To utilize the shoulders and chest

Circle both arms, reaching up above head, then out and down to complete circle. Breathe in as arms lift, out as they come down. Repeat 5 times.

135

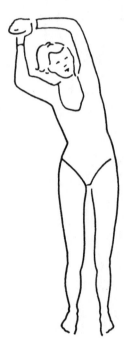

SIDE STRETCH
To stretch out the waist, back and sides and loosen the lower spine

Stand with feet hip-width apart. Raise both hands above head and clasp left wrist with right hand. Gently pull wrist to right side, stretching upwards and slightly over from the waist. Hold for 10 seconds. Repeat 5 times. Repeat on other side.

STRETCHES FOR STRENGTH & FLEXIBILITY

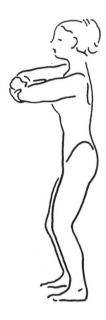

CHEST AND BUST FIRMER
To strengthen arms, shoulders, back and chest

Hold your wrists at shoulder-height in front of you. Grip as if pushing each hand towards the opposite elbow. Hold for 10 seconds, then release. Repeat 3 times.

137

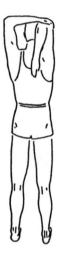

TRICEPS STRETCH
To stretch and tone the triceps and upper back

Raise arms and bend right elbow so that the right hand
rests on the upper back. Hold right elbow with left hand
and gently pull the right elbow in towards your head until
you feel a slight stretching sensation in the back of your
arm and across the upper back and shoulders. Hold for
10 seconds. Repeat 3 times and change arms.

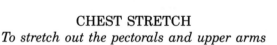

CHEST STRETCH
To stretch out the pectorals and upper arms

Stand with your feet apart. Clasp hands behind back; then
gently raise them, keeping your elbows slightly bent the
whole time. Hold for 8 seconds. Relax and repeat.

138

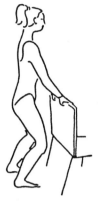

HALF SQUATS
To strengthen the thighs

With feet hip-width apart, and holding on to the back of
a chair for support, squat down, making sure that the angle
at the knee is never less than 90 degrees. Keep your upper
body upright. Return to the starting position. Repeat 10
times.

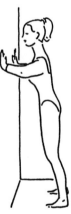

WALL PUSH-UPS
To strengthen and develop the arm, shoulder and chest
muscles

Stand about 3 feet from a wall. Raise arms to shoulder-
height and place on wall. Slowly bend arms as much as
you can to the count of 3. Then return to starting position
to the count of 3 and repeat 10 times.

139

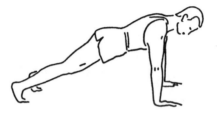

PUSH-UPS
To strengthen arms, shoulders, back and chest

Lie face down, palms flat beside shoulders and toes tucked under. Breathe in, then, breathing out, push up as far as possible. Breathe in and lower to a couple of inches above the floor. Repeat 5-10 times.

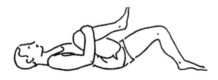

LOWER BACK STRETCH
To stretch out the hamstrings, inner thighs and back

Lie flat on back, knees bent, feet flat. Pull one knee towards you gently until you feel a slight stretch in the back of the thigh. Hold for 15-20 seconds. Repeat with other leg.

CURL-UPS
To strengthen stomach and back

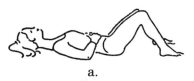

a.

a. Lie on back, knees bent, with feet and knees hip-width apart. Place hands lightly on stomach. Press your back to the floor.

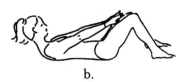

b.

b. Slowly curl up from the stomach and raise shoulders and head a couple of inches, reaching with both hands toward knees. Gently lower. Breathe out going up, and in going down. Repeat 5 times, pause, then repeat 5 times.

141

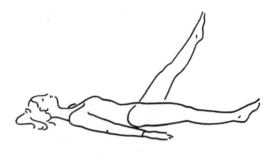

LEG LIFTS
To strengthen abdomen, thighs and lower back

Lie on your back, arms outstretched. Slowly raise then lower each leg alternately, counting 5 to raise, 5 to hold and 5 to lower. Don't arch your back. Repeat 5 times, relaxing between.

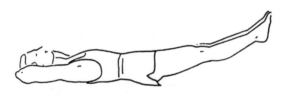

LEG RAISES
To strengthen abdomen, thighs and lower back

Lie on your back, legs together, arms behind your head. Keeping legs straight, raise feet gently from floor a few inches, keeping small of back pressed down on floor. Hold for 5-10 seconds. Repeat 5 times.

BACK PUSH-UP
To strengthen middle of back and shoulders and firm up
thighs and buttocks

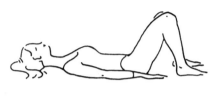

a.

a. Lie flat on floor, knees bent, arms by your side. Pull your stomach in and breathe deeply from abdomen for 10 seconds, keeping lower back pressed flat.

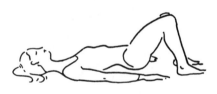

b.

b. Then lift buttocks off floor by contracting them and using your stomach muscles. Hold for 5 seconds. Repeat 5 times.

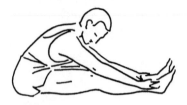

SITTING TOE TOUCHES
To stretch the inner thighs, spine, hamstrings, shoulders and back

Sit on floor, legs straight out in front, feet together, backs of knees touching the floor. Very slowly reach forward from the waist as far as is comfortable, clasping the calves, and keeping the spine and neck long. Hold for 10 seconds. Repeat 3 times.

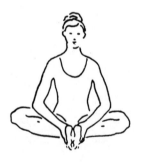

INNER THIGH STRETCH
To stretch out the groin area

Sit with the soles of your feet together and as close to you as is comfortable. Keep your back straight. Hold your ankles and press your knees downwards. Hold for 10 seconds; then release. Repeat 3 times.

144

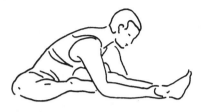

LOWER BACK STRETCH
To stretch out the lower back, and inside and back of thighs

Sit up with left leg straight and right leg bent. Gently
lean over the left leg from the hips until you feel a slight
stretching sensation down the back of the outstretched leg.
Hold for 10 seconds. Repeat 3 times, alternating legs.

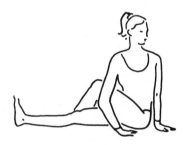

SPINAL STRETCH
To stretch out lower back and side of hip

Sit, legs outstretched. Place left foot over right leg, then
place left hand behind you and right hand across your body
for support. Slowly twist to left. Stretch body and turn
head gently to side. Do 3 twists, then change over legs;
right foot over left leg, and repeat exercise.

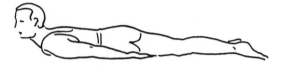

BACK STRENGTHENER
To strengthen the lower back

Lie face down on floor with hands under thighs. Gently lift head a couple of inches, hold and relax. Don't arch your back. Repeat 5 times.

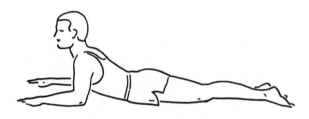

THE COBRA
To mobilize the spine and strengthen the back

Lie face down, palms flat on the floor at shoulder-height with elbows tucked into sides. Gently push up until you are resting on your elbows. Keep your spine and neck in line, still watching the floor so that you don't twist neck. Hold for 10 seconds, then relax. Repeat 5 times.

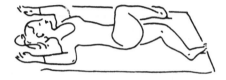

BACK STRETCH
To stretch out the center of the back, and tone and strengthen the thighs, buttocks, shoulders, arms and abdomen

Lie on back with knees bent and feet flat. Raise arms out to shoulder-height and bend at elbows so that the backs of the hands are flat on the floor. Don't arch your back. Bring your right leg over the left, lowering the knee towards the floor. Hold for 10 seconds. Repeat on other side.

147

COOL-DOWN STRETCHES

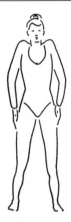

SHOULDER CIRCLES
To loosen and relax the neck, shoulders and back

Stand, arms at sides, with feet shoulder-width apart. Gently lift shoulders and move them backwards in a continuous rolling motion. Repeat 5 times, then repeat with a forward rolling motion.

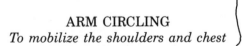

ARM CIRCLING
To mobilize the shoulders and chest

Circle both arms, reaching up above head, then out and down to complete circle. Breathe in as arms lift, out as they come down. Repeat 5 times.

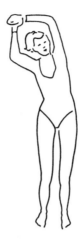

SIDE STRETCH
*To stretch out the waist, back and sides and loosen
the lower spine*

Stand with feet hip-width apart. Raise both hands above
head and clasp left wrist with right hand. Gently pull wrist
to right side, stretching upwards and slightly over from
the waist. Hold for 10 seconds. Repeat 5 times. Repeat on
other side.

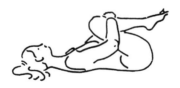

KNEE CLASP
To release tension in stomach and back

Lie with back flat on floor, legs together outstretched.
Breathing deeply from abdomen, pull knees toward chest
one by one. Breathe out, clasping knees and pressing lower
back down. Hold for 10 seconds.

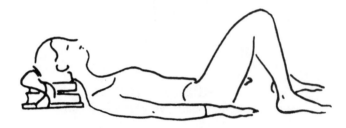

TOTAL RELAXATION

Lie flat on back, knees bent, arms at sides, and support the back of head with books piled to a height of about 4 inches. Breathe deeply from abdomen and concentrate on relaxing every part of the body. Start with the toes and say to yourself "my toes are completely and totally relaxing." Work up through the rest of the body: the legs, stomach, chest, back, shoulders, to the head, using the same relaxing words, but using your own version. A total relaxation session can last from 5 to 15 minutes or longer.

·5·

WALK AWAY FROM STRESS

Walk and be happy,
Walk and be healthy.

CHARLES DICKENS

Two of the main problems of living in modern Western society are:

1. Being tense, anxious and stressed
2. Sitting around much of the day (being sedentary).

This leads some people to the view that modern life itself is a disease, which expresses itself in obsessive work, anger, cynicism, fatigue, an inner hunger that nothing can fill, overeating, excessive smoking and alcoholism—often symptoms of dis-ease with oneself and the world.

Tension is something that we all feel from time to time—our muscles are wound up, our brain is overworked, we feel fatigued and overwrought. Tension is a symptom of anxiety, the "fight or flight" response of primitive survival behavior.

In primitive times danger often meant anxiety, and

151

anxiety provided the energy to respond effectively with "fight or flight." That was fine for primitive man, but the choice for modern man in industrialized Western civilization is not as simple. How can he choose between "fight or flight" if he feels cornered, ill-equipped and uncertain about which course of action to take.

We live in an age of uncertainty: an age of rapid change with increasing pressures and the need to survive. Some people call it the psychotoxic society where the chief protagonist in the drama is stress.

Stress is now considered to be the number-one killer in the Western world. In the United States, estimates for the combined cost to industry each year of stress-related absenteeism, low productivity, and medical insurance is said to be $75 billion. And surveys show that 75 to 90 percent of people visiting doctors suffer from stress-related problems.

These days, not only is work, divorce, retirement and bereavement stressful, but getting married we are told is also stressful. Taking vacations is stressful—even dieting, exercise and the quest for fitness are stressful.

We talk about "stress management." We attend stress relief classes, meditation centers, positive thinking classes. Some people take up juggling; others spend time in flotation tanks trying to relax.

The basis of most stress is anxiety and emotional conflict. Stressful conditions sooner or later translate into bodily symptoms causing tension, aching joints, headaches and backache, insomnia and depression.

Stress destroys essential vitamins and minerals and lowers the body's immune response. It triggers fatigue and leads to biochemical changes in our bodies. Unchecked, these biochemical changes can damage our heart and vascular system, resulting in high blood pressure, strokes and other diseases.

CAN WE AVOID STRESS?

How do we break away from stress, from "the thousand natural shocks that flesh is heir to" as Shakespeare put it?

We don't. We can no more avoid stress than we can avoid eating, drinking or breathing. Stress is part of life. And stress (good stress) can be motivating and stimulating. It is only a problem when it gets on top of us: when it is out of control (bad stress).

Bad stress is often associated with anxiety, fear, overwork, insomnia, boredom, grief and poor self-image. Taken to extremes it can lead to debilitating illness. Good stress, on the other hand, is encountered when we meet challenging situations (meeting new people, a job interview, making a public speech) or when we push ourselves to get things done.

Modern living is by its very nature fragmentary and specialized. The problem began with the Scientific Revolution in the 16th and 17th centuries. In order to understand the structure of Nature, man began to dissect everything that came under his control.

And then the problem developed further with the Industrial Revolution in the late 18th and early 19th centuries, when people left the land in increasing numbers to work in the towns. Division of labor often took away the satisfaction and personal worth felt by the individual craftsman and made him feel that he was no more than a cog in a machine.

Although these revolutions have helped put men on the moon and have given us the life-saving advances of modern medicine, on their negative side they have often left modern man in a state of alienation with himself, his neighbor and the society he lives in. Stress is only one expression of the loss of balance felt by modern man.

The philosopher Plato suggests in his famous allegory

that we are all like prisoners in a cave, and that what we take to be real are only shadows thrown upon the wall of the cave by a fire.

We spend too much time inside our heads; too much time inside buildings; too much time inside houses and cars. We need to get out: get outside of our heads, get outside of the artificial cocoons we have surrounded ourselves with, get out into the open air where the perspective is clear and we can see into the distance, beyond the windows and the four walls around us, and the people inside them.

Instead of trying to break away from stress what we should be doing is trying to neutralize its harmful effects. Like a tightrope walker, each day we tread the perilous road between good stress and bad stress. For some people it is not a problem; but for increasing numbers of people it is a problem—a dead end street with no way out. They lose their balance on the tightrope and fall off.

SEDENTARY MAN UNDER STRESS

Not only do we now have the psychotoxic society, but we have the hypokinetic society and hypokinetic disease: disease resulting from too little physical activity.

Dr. Hans Selye is the scientist who put the word "stress" into our scientific language. In his well-known experiment, he took ten sedentary laboratory rats and subjected them to blinding lights, electric shocks and incessant noise. In a month they were all dead. He took a further ten rats and exercised them regularly on a treadmill, then subjected them to the same stressful conditions. A month later they were all alive and thriving. Exercise had given them the psychological edge to cope with stress.

In human beings there is a paradox of exercise: as more

exercise is done, then more energy becomes available. The body seems to like being challenged; it moves into "overdrive," and it is this regular exercise that allows both human beings and animals to cope with stress.

However, as so many human beings in Western society are sedentary, it is hardly any wonder that their bodies are increasingly at the mercy of stressful conditions, cardio-vascular and respiratory disease and orthopedic problems. We would not treat a dog the way we treat ourselves. Imagine what Fido would be like if you only took him out for a walk once a week.

We have to break out of the routines and habits that hold us in their power and sap our vital energy. This is what the true meaning of exercise really is. It comes from the Latin word "ex-acere" meaning to break out from a shut-in state.

Some people try to relieve stress by playing games such as squash, golf, tennis or bowling; or they swim or take a vacation to get away from it all. All these activities no doubt lift the spirits, but the trouble with them all is that they are intermittent, anaerobic, start-stop activities. None of these activities has the stress-relieving quality of brisk, continuous, rhythmic walking.

Walking is a holistic experience. Walking disperses the ingrained patterns of physical inactivity and stress. Walking is a totally natural expression of the human body both physically and mentally.

WALKING—THE PERFECT EXERCISE

Walking normally we see the world at up to 3 miles an hour. But when we put our feet down for a brisk aerobic walk we increase our speed up to 3.5–4.0 miles an hour.

Our bodies are designed for action and movement—not

for sitting, standing, sauntering and strolling. As we walk, the spine flexes with each stride, then springs back again. Our feet work like the suspension on a car, the arched support of each foot absorbing the impact of weight as it makes contact with the road surface. Then as we begin to move, the forward pull of the torso becomes the engine to propel us forward under the force of gravity. With each stride first one, then the other leg swings out on its ball-and-socket hip joint as the muscles in the feet, legs, hips, back, shoulder and neck all work rhythmically together like the players in a symphony orchestra.

All of this is perfectly natural like the flight of a bird or the movement of a fish through water. Walking does not strain and pull the muscles and ligaments as jogging can; it does not overstretch and overdevelop the legs as cycling can. The body moves rhythmically through space in the way it was designed to do three million years ago.

Professor Owen Lovejoy, an anthropologist at Kent State University, made the following observation in *Scientific American* on walking and its place in man's development:

> Asked to choose the most distinctive feature of the human species, many people would cite our massive brain. Others might mention our ability to make and use sophisticated tools. A third feature also sets us apart: our upright mode of locomotion, which is found only in human beings and our immediate ancestors... The development of erect walking may have been a crucial initiating event in human evolution.

We used to believe that man had been walking upright for between one and two million years. Professor Lovejoy went on to suggest that upright walking could date back 3 million years and possibly some 8 or 10 million years, to the earliest hominids. Why then, after evolution has worked so hard to perfect the human body, is homo sapiens going out of its way to turn back the clock and undo all those years of fine tuning done by evolution?

A PSYCHO-PHYSICAL TONIC

It is brisk, aerobic walking that can break down the cycle of stress and tension that is the bane of life in the late 20th century. By the rhythmic action of the muscles, stress and tension are drained off and dissipated, and the body is restored to its natural state of equilibrium. It is this sense of rhythm that is described here by Tom Chetwynd in his book, *A Dictionary of Symbols:*

> Inner turmoil, conflict, confusion leads directly to walking...walking restores a sense of balance and brings an inner calm...is archetypally symbolic...the left foot alternates with the right, the conscious side with the unconscious side, between heart (the emotional life, the feminine side) on the left of the body and reason on the right, and so between the opposing pressures which caused the turmoil in the first place. The action of walking erect and balanced, like a vertical line, the world axis, can unite conscious and unconscious, mind and matter, in a way that thinking never can.

Walking is the perfect way to relax. You can use it to disperse tension or to prevent tension. Outside on the road, the mind and body find their own rhythm, not the rhythm imposed on them by circumstances. They are no longer playing second string to other discordant rhythms; they are on their own. Outside on the road it is a solo performance.

As you feel the rhythm and movement in your feet, calves, thighs, arms and shoulders, you will begin to let go, to truly let go and flow with it all. Your breathing will deepen naturally and become more regular and your circulation will respond as fresh oxygenated blood flows around your body.

Negative emotions will drain away while you walk. Problems that have been nagging away at your mind may be solved. The Greek philosopher Socrates used to talk about: "...the blessed fruit of the vine which reduces great disasters into small inconveniences." We can say the same about walking. Walking takes hold of the linear patterns of much of our daily thinking, and reorders them in a holistic way. Seemingly insoluble problems melt away during the continuous rhythmic flow of walking. Tension and stress become things of the past.

RHYTHMIC BREATHING

Walking is as natural as breathing and breathing is as natural as walking. To breathe is to live and without breath there is no life. Life is a series of breaths: from the first breath of the infant to the last gasp of the dying man.

We can exist for a time without eating; we can exist for a shorter time without drinking; but without breathing our life will be cut short after a few minutes. What really matters to us is the quality of our breathing, and it is here that we can make a significant contribution in assisting our mind and body to free themselves from tension and anxiety.

Although breathing deepens naturally as we walk, we may still be taking in less oxygen if we are breathing mainly from the chest area rather than using deep rhythmic breathing from the diaphragm. This is the type of breathing used in the practice of meditation and Yoga.

Efficient breathing through the nostrils pulls the air

deep into the lungs, expanding the lungs downward, and the lungs and chest outward. To breathe deeply, inhale by first moving your abdomen outwards. You will feel your stomach rise, then your upper abdomen, and finally your chest. Then breathe out by letting your stomach relax. It may feel strange at first, but this is the way that most of us breathe when we sleep.

Slow deep rhythmic breathing can double the volume of air you inhale with each breath, and together with brisk aerobic walking, it is the first step to attaining full relaxation and increased awareness. Deep rhythmic breathing will revitalize you. Muscles will relax and the mind will clear, as tension and stress are drained away and you let go totally.

As you increase your walking pace, you may want to try linking your breathing to it. For example: breathe in, counting (mentally) $1, 2, 3, 4, 5, 6, 7, 8$, one count to each step, making the inhalation extend over the eight counts. Then exhale slowly through the nostrils, counting as before - $1, 2, 3, 4, 5, 6, 7, 8$ - one count to each step. Rest between breaths and then continue at will. Experiment: you may find that counting to 4 or 6 or even 10 may suit you better. Counting breaths helps you to focus on a single idea, and it is an effective stress releaser. It is covered further in the next chapter under "Walking Meditation."

You may want to try what we call energy breathing. This really gets you going when you feel sluggish. Do the same exercise above, but instead of exhaling through the nostrils, exhale through the mouth: breathe in through the nostrils counting 1 to 8, then out through the mouth counting 1 to 8.

Another tension releaser is to get into a rhythmic stride and concentrate on relaxing each part of the body in turn. Start out by saying to yourself "my toes are relaxing...my feet are relaxing...my legs are relaxing..."

and so on up through your body until you reach the top of your head. Say to yourself "the tensions and troubles of the day are all draining out of my body...I feel totally at peace with myself and the world...I feel terrific."

THE ANSWER TO STRESS

By now you should be walking regularly for health, fitness and slimness; and you will have noticed the effect that walking has on helping you relax, whatever time of the day it is.

The body has its own rhythms, regulating temperature, hunger, mood, and alertness. It is these rhythms which explain why most people are sluggish early in the morning, and why they are much more alert later in the day. Body rhythms can be affected by many factors: food, drink, drugs, smoking, and lack of sleep. But the good news is that we can control our body rhythms (our body clocks) by brisk aerobic walking.

MORNING WALKS—Walk aerobically first thing in the morning for between 15 and 30 minutes to prepare yourself for the day ahead. Even if you only have time for a ten minute walk, you will experience immediately the relaxing effect of getting out of the house away from telephones, people, and the throb of civilization. You will feel your body "getting into gear" for the day as it takes in fresh supplies of oxygen and begins working like the efficient machine it is meant to be.

Walking first thing in the morning boosts your body temperature, makes you feel more alert and breaks those "early morning blues." But you must warm up thoroughly before walking, especially in the morning, and take it a little easier than usual—strolling for a few minutes before getting into a brisk stride.

160

AFTERNOON WALKS—Tension and anxiety often build up through the day, so lunchtime and afternoon walks can drain them off, leaving you feeling refreshed for the rest of the working day.

Instead of sitting around at lunchtime, go for a brisk aerobic walk for at least 20 minutes, then eat a light Walking Diet lunch. There is a lot of evidence to suggest that exercise depresses the appetite and helps with weight control.

EVENING WALKS—The evening may be the time that you choose to do your main aerobic walking, in which case it is better to walk before your evening meal to gain the maximum benefit from it. But if you have already put in the necessary aerobic miles for the day, you may want to use an evening walk to reflect on the day and use a quiet walk as a way of de-stressing.

Walking has a relaxing effect on the mind and it drains off the muscular tension in the body that has built up during the working day. After an evening walk you will be ready to retire to bed for a sound, uninterrupted night's sleep. There is evidence to suggest that walking in the evening may help insomnia.

WALKING BREAKS—Next time you stop for a coffee break, or stop to have a cigarette, change your mind and go for a ten minute walk instead. Not only will your body thank you for it—caffeine is a stimulant and increases tension, and nicotine is a toxin—but you will actually feel better for it.

MUSIC WHILE YOU WALK—Some people like to take a Walkman with them on their aerobic walks. They find that the rhythm of certain types of music helps them to walk at a steady pace and achieve a state of deep relaxation. Classical music, marches, swing, country, and pop music can all help dissolve stress.

The mind is a human instrument and physical and mental health can be affected by certain types of music. The composer Mendelssohn said: "Music cannot be expressed in words, not because it is vague but because it is more precise than words." Used with an aerobic walking schedule, music can help unlock the cycle of stress and produce a state of calm.

Experiments have shown that Baroque music (composed in the second half of the seventeenth and first half of the eighteenth centuries) can have a deep calming and relaxing effect on the mind.

Just remember that if you listen to music while you walk, then look where you are going. It may not be such a good idea to do it if you are walking in a busy urban area.

WALKING WITH OTHERS—Walking with a friend can help motivate you to build up a regular aerobic routine and can also help you to de-stress after a hard day's work. The continuous rhythmic effect of walking dissolves stress and clears the mind. It is only when the mind and body are fully relaxed in this way that problems are simplified and solutions present themselves.

It is often said that a problem shared is a problem halved. Talk through the problems of the day and look for creative solutions to them. People who have good friends to talk to don't usually need psychiatrists.

One research group has suggested that one reason many people give up exercising is because of marriage and family commitments. People with this problem should try walking. Walking is the easiest exercise of all to share with others. Walk with your spouse, your children, and your relatives. How many problems in the home, we wonder, could be solved simply by taking a walk. If you find yourself in conflict with your spouse, children or in-laws, then take them for a walk. Out there on the road, troubles dissolve, and you can find the time and space to put them into perspective.

Walk in the morning before tension become a problem, and walk at lunchtime to dispel the tensions of the morning. Walk in the early evening before dinner and walk before retiring to bed. The Dutch theologian Erasmus used to say: "Before supper walk a little; after supper do the same." Walk on your own or walk with others. Whatever the time of day, walk for the sheer joy and relaxation of walking. Whichever way you look at it, the best stress therapy is walking.

·6·

THE ART OF
WALKING

Afoot and light-hearted I take to the
open road,
Healthy, free, the world before me,
The long brown path before me leading
wherever I choose.

Henceforth I ask not good fortune, I
myself am good fortune,
Henceforth I whimper no more,
postpone no more, need nothing,
Done with indoor complaints, libraries,
querulous criticisms,
Strong and content I travel the open
road.

LEAVES OF GRASS,   WALT WHITMAN

There is a need for us all to renew ourselves from time to
time and take stock of who we are and where we are going.
There are many ways to do this. Some people turn to
organized religion and prayer, others to Eastern methods
such as yoga and Zen Buddhism. Yet others seek enlight-
enment in depth psychology and art.

Earlier in this book we introduced the Greek idea of
"diata," and suggested that health and fitness is about
much more than extreme diet and exercise routines; it is
in fact a whole way of life. We have looked in detail about

how to achieve the fit, healthy bodies and minds that we all desire. But life is surely about more than simply having a healthy mind in a healthy body.

"Know thyself," the Greek philosopher Socrates said. "If I am not myself, who else will be?" the walking philosopher and writer Thoreau said.

The longest journey we ever make is the journey within. We may use one of the more traditional methods to come to a greater realization of ourselves and discover a deeper meaning of life, or we may improvise our own methods using one or all of the above disciplines. The important thing is the realization that we need to make the journey if we are to be whole.

Some people use prayer, others use meditation and yoga techniques to prepare for the journey inward. The one thing that they all have in common is the need for total relaxation: a letting go of obsessive thoughts and all the clutter and confusion going on in the mind.

So where do we start?

"The way out is via the door." (Lao-Tse)

WALKING MEDITATION

Once you have discovered the benefits of aerobic walking for health, fitness and slimness, you will want to go further and discover the additional benefits provided by inner walking.

Inner walking is walking meditation, and it begins with relaxation and the feeling of letting go. Inner walking has nothing to do with goals or objectives. Use aerobic walking to get fit, improve your cardiovascular system and lose weight; use inner walking to encounter a deeper self-knowledge, greater concentration and serenity.

You can use walking meditation to break the pattern of

obsessive thoughts and tension. You can use it to center yourself inside your own experience and give yourself an overview of what is happening inside—what is really happening, not what you thought was happening. Walking meditation will give you control over your life.

How does it work?

There is a saying that the mind is like a drunken monkey. Think for a moment about the daily traffic of sounds going on inside your head, from the minute that you wake up to the minute that you go to bed. Think about the constant voice-over in your mind as a continuous sound track superimposed on an endlessly rolling film.

That is what the mind is like much of the time. And then think what it would be like to slow it all down and feel that it is you that is in control, and not the machinery that is controlling you.

The key to walking meditation is to keep your mind focused on what you are doing. You may be able to do this by simply walking for a while and letting the feeling of deep relaxation take over and provide the focus that you seek. Or you may want to use one of the traditional meditation methods to help you. You could try counting steps or counting breaths, or you could try using a mantra.

Counting your footsteps is a simple method to keep you in the here and now. You can count up to 10, 20, or a 100, either forwards or backwards, repeating it over and over. If that becomes a habit then try the following method:

1. Count your first seven steps.
2. With your next step, begin at 1 and count to 8.
3. Then with your next step, begin at 1 and count to 9.
4. Continue in the same way until you reach 12.
5. Repeat the sequence from the beginning as many times as you like.

Counting your breaths is another meditation which is easy to do. As you walk, count your exhalations up to 10 and begin again. If that becomes a habit, then instead of simply counting breaths you could pick out a lamp post or a tree a couple of hundred yards along the road and count your breaths until you get there. This helps to "anchor the mind" and focus awareness.

Using a mantra is another popular meditational practice. A mantra is a word or phrase that you can repeat to focus your awareness. "Om" is the most well known and is supposed to be "the eternal word," the basic sound of the universe. Any word or phrase that you can repeat to yourself as you walk along will do the job, but try to pick something that means something to you. Some people use words like "love" and "peace"—others use phrases such as "be still and know that I am God" or "love one another."

The easiest way to experience walking meditation is simply to concentrate on the body movements you make. Feel the weight of your heel as it makes contact with the ground, and the spring of your toe as the muscles in your leg propel you forward. Feel the rhythm of your arms and the movement of your head and all the sensory input that is going on. Feel the stillness in movement.

Meditation is about increased awareness, concentration and self-knowledge. Whether you relax naturally into it, or use one of the above methods, go with the flow. If you find your mind wandering, gently bring it back to the task of involving yourself more and more in it. Find a walking rhythm to suit you and stick with it.

Do the meditation as long as you need to. You are not working towards a goal. All you are trying to do is relax and center your mind. If you can do that, then you will be able to get away from the hurly burly of life any time you want to.

Another form of walking meditation is the thinking

walk: the walk to help you solve a problem. Writers, artists, philosophers and all types of creative people have used the thinking walk to help them with their work. They have spoken about the magical effect of walking and of how walking can act almost like a drug in its ability to free the mind and release its creative thought processes. The swinging, rhythmic action of walking drains off tension and anxiety and allows the mind to give total attention to the act of thinking, in a way that, for example, sitting in a chair thinking can never do. Try it. Next time you have a problem, take it with you for a walk and allow the action of the whole body and mind to sort it out for you. You will be amazed. Problems that seemed insoluble will simply melt away. And if you have personal problems you want to sort out with other people, ask them to join you for a walk. You will find that there are few problems that cannot be solved by taking a half-hour walk and talking things through.

Why should this be so? Walking, as we have already discovered, increases the supply of oxygen throughout our bodies. This is what makes walking an aerobic activity. And it is the increased supply of oxygen to the brain that stimulates our thought processes and enables us to see things more clearly and put them into perspective.

As well as the thinking walk, there is its opposite: the non-thinking walk—the Zen walk. During this walk, instead of consciously thinking through problems, the intention is to walk without thinking, to deliberately empty the conscious mind and allow the unconscious mind to take over and sort out the problem.

Try it out. Before your walk, go over in your mind the problem to be solved; then forget about it. Let the conscious mind relax, and let the problem go out of your mind. Don't set a time limit for a solution; the solution will come in its own good time. The unconscious mind will go on working in the background, and you will find that the answer to the problem will arise unexpectedly. It may be during the next walk you take, or the next day even. It does not matter when.

This type of problem-solving is creativity by "serendipity" —making discoveries that you are not consciously searching for, that happen by chance or accident. During the writing of this book we would often use either the thinking walk or the Zen walk to solve a particular writing problem, or to get going again when we were stuck. A brisk walk has often provided the solution to the problem in hand and allowed us to get going again.

RHYTHMS OF CHANGE

The conductor Sir Thomas Beecham said that music frees us from the tyranny of the conscious mind. Walking can have the same effect. The rhythmical effect of walking has a musical quality about it, and it is the measured beat of the right foot alternating with the left that helps to break down the negative patterns of inactivity and stress.

Walking frees us from the tyranny of the conscious mind; it helps us to look inside ourselves, to see ourselves clearly, away from the noise and distractions of modern living. Inner walking is a natural therapy which promotes a sense of peace and rhythm that we all need in our lives.

Rhythm is all around us: it pervades the Universe and the natural world. Modern physics sees matter as "being in a continuous dancing and vibrating motion whose rhythmic patterns are determined by the molecular, atomic and nuclear structures" (Fritjof Capra, *The Tao of Physics*). Some mystics, philosophers and poets also see the material world in the same way: as a dynamic universe that moves, vibrates, and dances. When we walk we move, vibrate, and dance with it.

The composer Gustav Mahler tells the story that he was once stuck in the middle of writing a new symphony. He was stuck for weeks. No matter how hard he worked, the notes did not come. Then one day he was being rowed across a lake. Suddenly, the rhythm and movement of the oars through the water created rhythms in his own mind and the notes for the opening of the next movement came to him.

Walking can be like this. With practice, once you get into a rhythm and really begin to relax and let go, walking can stimulate a meditational state similar to the deep meditational states of yoga and other disciplines.

I walk, therefore I am. I use inner walking to be with myself: to get away from the noise and distractions of everyday life. Out there on the road the mind suddenly clears. It is lifted out of the confused chatter that often goes on inside, and it sees as if for the first time, like a child.

WHO WERE THE INNER WALKERS?

Philosophers, poets, writers, musicians, and creative people of all types have been enthusiastic walkers—and for good reason. George Trevelyan, who wrote the classic *History of England*, said of walking, "I never knew a man go for an honest day's walk for whatever distance, great or small...and not have his reward in the repossession of his soul."

Aristotle, who was known for the Peripatetic school of philosophy, would discourse with his students while walking around the grounds of the Academy. Emmanuel Kant walked every afternoon, and Rousseau said of his walks, "Never have I thought so much, never have I realized my existence so much, I have been so much alive." Wordsworth, Shelley, Keats, Coleridge and de Quincey were all inveterate walkers. It was estimated by Wordsworth's friends that during the course of his life he walked 185,000 miles in the English Lake District, which inspired him to "see into the heart of things" and to write about:

A presence that disturbs me with the joy
Of elevated thoughts; a sense sublime
Of something far more deeply interfused,
Whose dwelling is the light of setting suns,
And the round ocean, and the living air,
And the blue sky, and in the mind of man:
A motion and a spirit, that impels
All thinking things, all objects of all thought,
And rolls through all things.

The modern Welsh poet R. S. Thomas has written of a similar feeling about walking in his poem, "The Moor."

It was like a church to me.
I entered it on soft foot,
Breath held like a cap in the hand.
It was quiet.
What God was there made himself felt,
Not listened to, in clean colors
That brought a moistening of the eye,
In movement of the wind over grass.

There were no prayers said. But stillness
Of the heart's passions—that was praise
Enough; and the mind's cession
Of its kingdom. I walked on,

Simple and poor, while the air crumbled
And broke on me generously as bread.

Dickens, Samuel Johnson, Boswell, Ruskin and Jane Austen all used their walks to free the creative mind. Beethoven and Mozart both took to the woods to discover their own "creator spiritus." Would Beethoven's *Pastoral Symphony* exist but for his walks in the Vienna woods? Would Mozart have given us *The Marriage of Figaro* if he had not sought inspiration in the open air? Not only men of genius, but ordinary people have been discovering for centuries that walking has a special quality about it.

Inner walking frees us from the tyranny of the conscious mind and lets the intuitive mind breathe.

THE INTUITIVE MIND

No one really knows how intuition works, but split brain research in recent years has given us a clue. Researchers have discovered that each side of the brain, the right and the left, processes information in its own way. Although the brain as a whole works together, one side or the other tends to predominate for a specific task.

Our left brain is verbal, objective, logical, analytical, linear, and conscious, whereas our right brain is non-verbal, subjective, intuitive, holistic, spatial, and unconscious. The problem for many of us in Western society is that we tend to be left brain dominant. We live in a society which values masculine, objective, analytical skills at the expense of feminine, subjective, intuitive skills.

If we are not careful, it is easy to become trapped and blindered in our own rational, linear thought patterns. We go on day after day in the same old way, often unhappy with our lot, but not knowing how to change it. We become stuck on a giant treadmill that turns forever without stopping.

The great Swiss psychologist, Carl Jung, summed up the modern Western way of thinking when he said that "we think with our tongues."

We need to give the right brain a chance. We need to free the intuitive mind. We need to let go and relax, for this has always been the first step in seeking the wholeness that we lack. You could say that we need something to inspire us. Inspire means literally "breathe into." We need to let go, relax, and let the intuitive mind breathe into us its spirit. We need to walk.

As you progress with inner walking and walking meditation, you will experience moments when you feel that everything suddenly becomes clear. At such moments life is filled with a significance which it normally lacks.

Inner walkers have described the feeling as follows:

> When I am alone, as it were, completely myself...walking after a good meal...ideas flow best and most abundantly. Whence and how they come, I know not; nor can I force them.
>
> WOLFGANG AMADEUS MOZART

> I can see the whole of it at a single glance in my mind...All the inventing and making goes on in me in a beautiful strong dream. But the best of all is the hearing of it all at once.
>
> WOLFGANG AMADEUS MOZART

> As I went along, thinking nothing in particular, only looking at things around me and following the progress of the seasons, there would flow into my mind, with sudden and unaccountable emotion, sometimes a line or two of verse, sometimes a whole stanza at once.
>
> A. E. HOUSMAN

JOURNEYS IN INNER TIME

There are few times when we are really alone with ourselves. We are always too busy. We say that we never have time. And yet we make time for almost everything else: eating, drinking, working, making love, entertainment and sleeping.

Time seems to be an elusive element in our lives which tends to get out of control, and if we are not careful it ends up controlling us. Time measures change: change between one hour and the next, one day and the next, and so on. In the short run we talk about having no time, losing time, spending time. In the long run, as the great economist Maynard Keynes said, we are all dead.

And yet despite the fact that time can be elusive and can appear to control us, there are times, rare occasions, when we catch a glimpse of something greater, more meaningful—times when we are totally alive and whole. It can happen listening to a piece of music, reading a poem, watching a film, falling in love, staring at the stars. On such occasions we become unaware of time. We talk about time "standing still." Certainly time slows down, and we become unconscious of it.

We have all experienced the feeling of time distortion. Waiting for a bus or train, we are conscious that time is passing very slowly: five minutes can seem like 20. And yet when we become fully absorbed in something that interests us, we experience the opposite: an hour can seem like ten minutes.

This is because time, clock time, is a phenomenon of the conscious left brain. Waiting for a train, we are still carrying around with us all the "mental baggage" of the day: we may be tense, angry, even fearful. Time drags. But when we do something that fully absorbs us, we let go of

175

all the "mental baggage" and relax. It is only then, when we fully relax and let go, that time appears to stand still and life becomes more meaningful.

Unless you are an ardent jogger, 20 minutes of jogging may seem endless to you. You go out all geared up to get fit, but the effort required is too great. You are anchored in your conscious mind. You are anxious for results. Time drags.

Walking, either brisk aerobic walking or inner walking, can produce the opposite effect. You can walk for 20 minutes and it can seem like five. You can walk for one hour and it can seem like 20 minutes. Time does not drag; you lose track of time. You are in another dimension.

To understand time we need to grasp that there are three different kinds of time, and that we live constantly in three separate time zones.

There is social time which we can also call clock time: experienced time, time that is measured in minutes, hours, days, and weeks; time which we organize our lives by in Filofaxes and train schedules. Time for birth, growth and death.

There is cosmic time, or Nature time, which we experience as the infinite: the expanding universe, the 15 million years back to the Big Bang; the seasons and evolution.

And there is inner time. Inner time has nothing to do with clocks, calendars or social conditioning. It has nothing to do with the expanding universe or the seasons. Inner time is a time when we are alone. It is a time when we are truly with ourselves, when we can reflect and remember just who we are.

Inner time is what inner walking is all about. We leave behind the weight of clock time and social time and on the road we find ourselves, and discover the inscape of our deepest selves.

The story is told of a Zen master who was invited to

give a lecture to his students. The students assembled in a great rectangular hall and sat waiting patiently for the master to arrive. Outside it was raining and the only sound inside the hall was the sound of the rain tapping against the roof.

When the master arrived, he sat down before them, and he too waited patiently, listening quietly to the sound of the rain tapping against the roof.

Suddenly the rain stopped. The master got up and asked the students to follow him outside. The students eagerly followed the master as he left the building and began to stride briskly away from them towards the hills in the distance, as though rapt in a trance. The students had to hurry, for the master had long legs and he was already starting to leave them behind.

They took a circular route across the hills, and then down through some woods near a stream, before returning to the great rectangular hall. During the journey, no one had spoken. And no one could remember how long they had walked or how far.

The students assembled again in the hall, and the master sat before them. They waited and waited, anxiously expecting the master to speak and impart his wisdom to them.

After a time the master quietly stood up; he said that the lecture was over, and left.

The sound of the rain needs no translation

Zen saying

THE ROAD AHEAD

Not I, not any one can travel that road for you,
You must travel it for yourself.

WALT WHITMAN

177

So what do we find on these inner walks, you might ask? If we knew the answer to that question we would know the answer to the meaning of existence itself. We walk to be alone: to discover something about ourselves that we did not know, or we had forgotten. We walk simply to be ourselves—whatever that means, for your inner walks will tell you something different to mine.

I can only tell you that the days when I do no inner walking I feel incomplete, as if something is missing. As much as possible, I try to keep my mind focused during the day on making sure that nothing prevents me from getting out and enjoying my inner walks.

Inner walking works not only while you walk, but it carries over to affect the whole of the rest of your life: your relationships, your work, your hopes and your dreams.

There is an ancient legend of a man who traveled the entire world in search of buried treasure. After a lifetime's search he returned tired and weary to his home village where a child pointed out to him that the treasure he had been seeking was inside himself.